STEROIDS
Keys to Life

STEROIDS
Keys to Life

Rupert F. Witzmann

Translated by Rosemarie Peter
Foreword by Hans Selye

VNR VAN NOSTRAND REINHOLD COMPANY
NEW YORK   CINCINNATI   ATLANTA   DALLAS   SAN FRANCISCO
LONDON   TORONTO   MELBOURNE

This book was originally published under the title *Schlüssel des Lebens* by Rupert Witzmann © 1977 by Verlag Fritz Molden.

Translation by Rosemarie Peter

Van Nostrand Reinhold Company Regional Offices:
New York   Cincinnati   Atlanta   Dallas   San Francisco

Van Nostrand Reinhold Company International Offices:
London   Toronto   Melbourne

Library of Congress Catalog Card Number: 80-19388
ISBN 0-442-29590-1

Manufactured in the United States of America

Published by Van Nostrand Reinhold Company
135 West 50th Street, New York, N.Y. 10020

Published simultaneously in Canada by Van Nostrand Reinhold Ltd.

15   14   13   12   11   10   9   8   7   6   5   4   3   2   1

Library of Congress Cataloging in Publication Data

Witzmann, Rupert, 1919–
   Steroids.

   Translation of Schlüssel des Lebens.
   Bibliography: p.
   Includes index.
   1. Steroid hormones. 2. Metabolic regulation.
I. Title.
QP572.S7W5713   612'.405   80-19388
ISBN 0-442-29590-1

Foreword

I was very glad to receive an invitation from Dr. Rupert Witzmann to write an Introduction to his book on *Schlüssel des Lebens,* and was especially happy to see that this informative book will be published in my native city of Vienna by one of its best known and respected companies, Molden Verlag.

But it is not only for sentimental reasons that I am pleased to learn of the publication of Dr. Witzmann's book. The more I travel around the world, lecturing on stress and talking to people from all walks of life, the more I am convinced that the general public wants to understand exactly what happens to them physically when they are under stress. Thus it seems to me a commendable goal to explain the steroids and their function to the layman in language easily understandable to all.

Although my specialty is stress per se, my interest in the steroids goes back even further. When I was 21 years old I presented a paper on the toxic effect of vitamin D, a steroid derivative, to the "Verein deutscher Ärzte in Prag," an event that undoubtedly made a deeper impression on me than on the learned men in the audience. That paper was published a few months later in the *Medizinische Klinik.* The work supporting this article got me interested in the closely related steroid hormones, and from then on my fascination with this group of compounds grew. In 1943 I published a four-volume encyclopedia on their chemistry and pharmacology and, although this ambitious enterprise achieved only very modest success, I learned that the steroids were a vast and intricate field of science that could provide scientists with questions to study for years to come.

Even if my main interest shifted from the steroids to the stress concept, I remained faithful to this subject throughout my long career, for I am still trying to decipher the mysteries of the steroids in my work on resistance to stress and the diseases of stress, or "diseases of adaptation," which are largely dependent upon naturally occurring steroids.

However, the complexities of the steroids should not frighten away the general public who might like to learn more about this aspect of science.

Rather, the intricacies should provide a challenge to those who enjoy trying to figure out the mysteries of Nature. In my own first German book, *Stress beherrscht unser Leben,* I wrote the following introductory note:

> Dieses Buch ist all jenen gewidmet, die sich
> nicht fürchten, den Stress eines ausgefüllten
> Lebens in vollen Zügen zu geniessen und nicht
> so naiv sind, anzunehmen, dass dies ohne
> geistige Bemühung geschehen könne.

These words, written about stress, apply equally to the broader field of steroids in general.

Consequently Dr. Witzmann's book is not to be read merely as entertainment. It has enormous instructive value and is worth the effort of concentration for those who want to extend their education to the sciences, even without any special training. It is evident from the amount of literature cited that Dr. Witzmann has spent a great deal of time and effort going through all pertinent publications in this field. He is not satisfied with presenting his readers with a superficial, elementary outline, but goes deeply into specific aspects of the steroid question. One of the great fascinations about this book is that he manages to put together a panoramic view of the steroids—which, after all, occupy a key position in life—while at the same time exploring their particular role in adaptation and resistance to various forms of stress. The reader is given both an overview of the picture in its entirety and a glimpse at the specific functions of the steroids.

This is a gigantic task, and Dr. Witzmann has managed to reach his goal in a manner that is scientifically sound and comprehensible to all. I wish this book the success it well deserves in all German-speaking countries.

Hans Selye, C.C.
M.D., Ph.D., D. Sc.
President, International
Institute of Stress

Preface

Our desire to learn more about ourselves and to benefit from this knowledge has advanced biological research to its present state. Yet the average citizen, toward whom this Cyclopean effort is directed, does not stand a chance, should he be foolhardy enough to try to learn from scientific publications what is being done in his behalf in thousands of laboratories all over the world. It is to this interested layman, a hundred times frustrated yet undaunted, that I dedicate this book.

In writing this book, I needed stimulation and assistance. I received both in conversations with Adolf Butenandt, Jerome Conn, E. Dane, H. Dannenberg, Charles Huggins, Peter Karlson, Feodor Lynen, Russel Marker, Tadeusz Reichstein, Leopold Ruzicka, Hans Selye, G. Thorn, and many others to whom I wish to express my gratitude. My special thanks are due to Adolf Windaus, whose name is inseparable from the steroids. His lectures at Göttingen laid within me the foundation for this book.

In regard to the American edition, I would like to thank Rosemarie Peter for her work which went far beyond the usual scope of a translation. Her judicious assistance has been an asset.

Acknowledgments

In the interest of maximum lucidity, the graphic illustrations, all newly drawn, are loosely modeled after standard, internationally accepted representations. The following is a representative list of sources which are gratefully acknowledged: C. Clegg/Mech. Horm. Act.; L. Fieser/Steroids; Geigy; W. Holland/Mol. Pharm.; P. Karlson/Biochem.; C. H. Li/Growth Horm.; C. Villee/Act. Ster. Horm.; R. Williams/Text. Endocr.

1. PICTURE CREDITS

Fig. 2-1. Picture Archives of the Austrian National Library, Vienna; Fig. 2-2. Picture Archives of the Austrian National Library, Vienna; Fig. 2-3. Picture Archives of the Austrian National Library, Vienna; Fig. 3-1. from Stockinger and Kerjaschki (adapted from Cepaldi); Fig. 3-2. Institute for Micromorphology and Electronmicroscopy (Prof. Dr. Leopold Stockinger), Vienna; Fig. 3-4. Picture Archives of the Austrian National Library, Vienna; Fig. 3-14. Ernst Böhm, Ludwigshafen; Fig. 3-30. Associated Press; Fig. 3-32. Picture Archives of the Austrian National Library, Vienna; Fig. 3-33. Picture Archives of the Austrian National Library, Vienna; Fig. 3-37. Picture Service, Burda-Verlag; Fig. 3-45. Archives of Prof. Hans Selye; Fig. 3-46. Studio Countess Irmgard v. Schwerin, Westmount; Fig. 3-54. Institute for Micromorphology and Electronmicroscopy (Prof. Dr. Leopold Stockinger), Vienna; Fig. 3-55. Urban & Schwarzenberg, Vienna; Fig. 5-1. Picture Archives of the Austrian National Library, Vienna (by permission from Photopress, Zurich); Fig. 6-6. Dr. H. Frost, Munich; Fig. 6-13. Selecta-Verlag, Munich.

2. COLOR PLATES

Toni Angermayer, Holzkirchen, W. Germany (1, 3 and 9, top and bottom); Burkard Kahl, Stuttgart (4, top and bottom); Heinz Löffler, Vienna (7 and

11); Helga Meseck, Vienna (13, top and bottom); Hans Pfletschinger, Ebersbach/Fils, W. Germany (14); Searle, Lausanne (5); Selecta-Verlag, Munich (16, top); Spanish Tourist Office (2); Stern, Hamburg (12, top and bottom); Reinboth, R. (10).

Contents

STEROIDS
Keys to Life

1. The Reason for Writing this Book

Never before did so few know so much
and so many so little . . .

The initial development went quite unnoticed: Modern research, having discovered and invented synthetics, antibiotics, computers, and much, much more that was considered progress, grew weary of these superficial matters and began to search for underlying truths, for the space beyond the stars, for the ultimate origin of matter, for the laws that govern the evolution of life.

Actually, a magnificent renaissance of philosophy was initiated by the theory of relativity and nuclear research and, after World War II, took possession of the science of life itself. Man started to ask about the "how" of life, instead of the "why" which he would never discover.

However, to the extent to which applied research was left behind, difficulties began to arise. The closer one approached the envisioned goals, the more research lost the clarity required for it to become an object of general interest. It began to isolate itself. Yet, isolation was not the only danger.

In order to cope with new problems, new specialties had to be created which like a Hydra, daily brought forth new disciplines and lost sight of the original goals. Today, the existence of millions of scientific publications overwhelms the most outstanding experts. This brings to mind the Sorcerer's Apprentice and suggests that, some day soon, all living researchers will have to spend their time doing nothing but passing on existing knowledge to subsequent generations:

. . . . And what there is to conquer
has already been discovered
Once or twice or several times. . . .

There is only the fight to recover
what has been lost
And found and lost again and again.

(T. S. Eliot, *Four Quartets*)

Dissatisfaction with the current state of affairs is not limited to the scientific community. Countercultures develop with their prophets and make it their business to question the validity of research as such. It has become fashionable to doubt—fashionable to sport nihilism like a lapel button. Is it any wonder?

It may have been 30 or 40 years ago that the educated layman read with interest (even if he did not understand all the details) how butadiene polymerizes or how the constitution of indigo was revealed. And the results, the material that came from the retorts, could be comprehended and touched, understood and used: india rubber, aniline dyes, the first chemotherapeutic substances. Today, however, one reads that a Nobel Prize was awarded for the "Elucidation of the Cyclic 3, 5–AMP Mechanism" or the "Stereo-structure of Cyclic Hydrocarbons," and one has no understanding of the whys and wherefores. One attempts to follow some shop talk about steroids and, upon hearing that "the buffer for the extraction of the AS-factor consists of 0.01 M NaN_3," one concludes with Socrates that "I was, by nature, entirely unsuited for this type of investigation." Thus the gap between the few who know, and the many who do not, becomes even larger.

There is yet another reason for this. Scientists all too easily yield to the temptation to awe the layman with their arrogant jargonizing and, consequently, reinforce his reluctance to inform himself about the increasingly less comprehensible developments of science.

However, there is no reason for such arrogance. While scientists have been in danger of losing themselves on the periphery of the abstract, the basic attitude in the Western world has returned to a focus on life and our place in it and is eagerly seeking to relate *to man* the exponentially expanding development of science. This is a great accomplishment of the layman, and he deserves gratitude for it. That his endeavor has not led to success but to frustration, cannot be blamed on him alone. The previously mentioned difficulties, such as the excessive specialization of science, the inability of the knowledgeable to communicate, and probably also—at least partially—the layman's inadequate education in science, are all at fault. However, these problems are not insurmountable.

In order to counteract excessive specialization, it is sufficient simply to step back once in a while and, immediately, great complexes will become discernible in the distance. The steroids, in terms of their significance for life, certainly represent such a complex, and this book is meant to facilitate "stepping back," so that the various inter-relationships can be recognized.

There is no doubt that such a field can be presented in its entirety in a generally comprehensible manner, although there are those who may turn up their noses at the necessary simplifications. This book, however, was written not for the expert, but for my neighbor who contemplates the caterpillars while watering his roses, for my minister, my family, and perhaps even my family physician who finished medical school 20 years ago.

The final objection, that the layman lacks the necessary basic knowledge, may be the most serious one. He alone can disprove it. It is true that the road to understanding has become more difficult than it was at the time of the "Microbe Hunters" or the "Men against Death." The material has become more intractable but by no means impossible to understand. In the twenties, nuclear physics, which had been an extremely esoteric field, encountered a public entirely unprepared for it in terms of scientific background. Nevertheless, thanks to Bohr's planetary model of the atom, the principles of nuclear physics and, especially, its significance are generally understood today. Similarly, the steroids represent a new kind of complex appearing on the horizon of our knowledge, this time in the field of biology. It too seems incomprehensible at first. However, if the layman truly wants to understand what is going on, he must be willing, occasionally, to wrestle with a few concepts which he may not have encountered at school. Just as, years ago, we had to learn the meaning of electron, proton and neutron, today such terms as protein molecule, steroid molecule and hormone blocker must be included in our lifelong learning process.

Daily adaptation of our education to the preveailing state of science is one of the necessities of our times. It is inevitable if we want progress (a word I use with caution), yet it is not without its problems. The fact that my daughters are more proficient than I am in vector calculation does not perturb me, since this is a question of fashionable variations of a procedure otherwise familiar to me. However, that they know more than I do about plutonium, or about the constitution of my country, does bother me since these are areas of concern to me where the knowledge I once acquired is outdated.

The situation is similar in the field of biology. Much of the information accumulated during those happy years, when we laid the—as we believed—unshakable foundation of our education, has become obsolete. In some cases, only the emphasis has shifted and the old knowledge is as good as the new. Often, however, the new is really new, and we must know it in order to understand what goes on every day, right in front of our eyes, on the frontiers of biological research.

Mastery of this new knowledge makes no greater demand on one's intelligence than figuring out the Munich mass transit fares. He who does not lose confidence or close his mind to the strange sounds of a few basic terms will—while believing himself helplessly adrift in the boundless ocean of information—unexpectedly come upon some rock formations breaking through the surface, which suggest the existence of a mountain range at the bottom of the ocean. This mountain range represents the unchanging principles of life, valid from its beginning in the Precambrian era until the death of the last bacterium on earth.

Among all the chance occurrences in life, which at first confuse us, we have learned to seek the basic, the primary, the inevitable, associated with the concept of life on this planet. A few of these rock formations are already visible. First, there was the secret of the organic materials, which it was believed only "life" could produce, until Wöhler showed, in 1828, how urea can be synthesized.

Then, for many years, proteins remained the great riddle. Finally, a second rock formation appeared when it was found that only 20 amino acids can produce all the proteins that ever existed on this earth. Chemists, using this knowledge to synthesize proteins (which, again, it had been believed could be produced only by a living substance), then began to survey this second rock formation as well.

Later on, more and more rock formations appeared, among them the largest one: Since it was found that all amino acids used by nature for protein synthesis rotate polarized light to the left only, whereas normal synthesis yields a mixture of dextrorotatory and levorotatory components, it was suspected that all proteins not only were related but also had come from the same workshop—in the dinosaur as in man—and that their synthesis was always based on the same mechanism. This thought led to the discovery of the genetic code. It showed that there actually existed, in the truest sense of the word, a gigantic blueprint from which one could summon the many thousands of protein enzymes that decided the way in which an egg cell would develop. However, who made the decision, or how the summoning was done, was unknown.

Then, about 50 years ago, an additional peak emerged from the ocean, but no one could guess at that time that it too would turn out to be part of a huge underwater rock formation. A number of powerful active substances had been discovered which, strangely enough, all belonged to a rare chemical group called steroids. Over the years, more and more substances of this group were found and, gradually, it began to dawn on scientists that nature's repetitively monotonous use of the same complicated core structure could no longer be considered an accident and that, perhaps, they had found another rock formation. However, its significance was not recognized at the time.

The road from the first discovery of the steroids, via their isolation, to their magnificent application in medicine, as well as the insights gained along the way, makes for an extraordinary story. Steroid research started in ancient times and ended its first chapter during the early twentieth century. By that time, almost all the clinical symptoms resulting from steroid defects in the human body had been discovered, but without insight into their underlying cause. This was the era of keen observers, naturalists and doctors. However, lacking the necessary technical developments, they were unable to recognize the common steroid nature of these diseases and to perceive all the diverse symptoms, accumulated over 2000 years, as parts of a greater whole.

The year 1903 marks the beginning of the second epoch, when a young chemist became involved in the study of nonsaponifiable fats for a reason which, in retrospect, can only be explained as a stroke of genius: he simply assumed that he was dealing with an important class of substances. He developed the methods necessary for working with these difficult substances and, with two or three other researchers from Germany and the United States, formed the "Gentlemen's Club" of steroid research—a little esoteric, a little senseless at that time, and perhaps also a little snobbish. Then the great discoveries of the twenties occurred, and the whole world sent its young scientists to the small Hanoverian university town of Göttingen. Over a period of 20 years, the Gentlemen's Club had managed to isolate almost all the important steroids, to elucidate their structure, and to reveal an unexpected connection between the hormones and the cardiac-active digitalis poisons, the bile acids, and cells' building materials, and vitamin D. It was the great adventure of the thirties which would never be repeated.

What followed then was the practical application of the results—the era of therapy. By means of the new active substances, one learned to perform miracles, turned invalids into healthy people, induced deficiency and excess conditions as nature had never known them, saved hundreds of thousands of children from rickets, and created the contraceptives which will probably have a decisive influence on the fate of mankind.

The technical epoch followed. The necessity of providing huge quantities of corticoids automatically started a race for raw materials that was reminiscent of the times of india rubber. Simultaneously, laboratories all over the world proceeded to improve on nature. Scientists examined the active spectrum of the hormones for unknown areas, hoping to isolate individual wavelengths, to amplify some and attenuate others. To stay with our analogy, the rock formation had been found and was being surveyed. A few divers ventured somewhat below the ocean surface, but no one had caught a glimpse of the mountains yet.

That only happened in the fifth period; the depths of the ocean were still dark, and help was needed from molecular biology before the outlines of the mountain range could become discernible. Then, one saw something marvelous: the steroids had provided us with the key to the genetic code which could be used to influence protein synthesis in the cell and, consequently, the fate of the whole individual. However, that is a long story.

To follow this story does not require a degree in medicine or chemistry, although we will mention a few facts about them now and then, since there is nothing at all sinister about chemistry—least of all about steroid chemistry. Years ago, in order to grasp the principle of the atomic bomb, it was adequate to learn that according to Bohr's model of the atom, there were electrons orbiting around protons and neutrons. Similarly, to understand steroid chemistry, it is sufficient to know that there are carbon atoms (C) which have arms (or valences) by means of which they hold on to one another in order to form chains. And, since each of these carbon atoms is endowed with four arms, two of them remain free to reach for additional atoms, preferably the one-armed hydrogen atoms (H). Five or six carbon atoms tend to form a ring, which is then called cyclopentane or cyclohexane, respectively, and in which each carbon atom holds on to two hydrogen atoms. This is illustrated in Fig. 1–1. To save time, one can simply draw a pentagon or hexagon, as shown in Fig. 1–2. A steroid, then, is simply any substance whose core consists of a skeleton comprising three cyclohexanes and one cyclopentane (see Fig. 1–3).

For the time being, one may picture this molecule with its 17 linked carbon atoms as a small, flat disc. Taking one good look at this esthetically beautiful formation will enable one forever to recognize a steroid without knowing anything else about chemistry. Certainly, the various steroids must somehow differ from one another, but this is easily accomplished. All it requires is that the hydrogen atoms, originally linked to the carbon atoms, be replaced by two-armed oxygen atoms (O) or by additional carbon atoms. How this

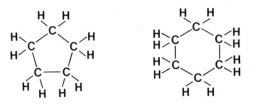

Fig. 1–1.

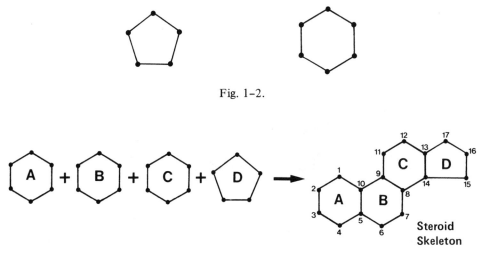

Fig. 1-2.

Fig. 1-3.

occurs will occasionally be mentioned in this book, and the reader can remember such material, or forget it, as he chooses.

We, however, shall not let this keep us from following with suspense the greatest attack on a single group of substances that the world has ever seen. From this, we will learn about the glittering opalescence of the sex hormones, the therapeutic miracle of cortisone, and the potency of the cardiac poisons. We will witness, step by step, how nature's secrets are wrested from her, how she is even surpassed and how, nevertheless, we must finally remain within the limits imposed by her.

2. Rocks Protruding from the Ocean Surface

For thousands of years, man had been on the trail of the great steroids—cholesterol, the bile acids, the cardiac glycosides, the hormones—and their effects. About 400 B.C., the father of medicine considered the troublesome gallstones worthy of being included in his Hippocratic oath. *Fel tauri desiccata,* dried ox bile, had been used as a bile-promoting medication since time immemorial; and the active substances of the sea onion, or squill, and the purple foxglove were used by both ancient Egyptians and Nero's physician to cure the deadly dropsy. This is to say nothing of the sex hormones, whose effects have been like a red thread running through the existence of living creatures.

Of course, no one had guessed that all these substances belonged together, that they all expressed nature's will to control life on this planet, and that the same group of substances was behind all these diverse effects. Man had held the parent substance in his hands as gallstones, without recognizing the connection, and thrown it away like a peasant finding a lump of uranium in his fields.

This was only partially a result of a lack of the technical prerequisites for recognizing the common steroid nature of these substances. Rather, in a more fundamental sense, it had something to do with man's not being ready to acknowledge the existence of substances which produced these effects. Of course, colic was caused by gallstones. However, the eminently more important question of whether or not there was a substance which, for instance, controlled reproduction, had never been raised, even by the ancient Greeks. Those same men who discussed the difficult subject of innate ideas, and had already concluded that the world must consist of atoms, had never questioned their own identity. For countless generations, it had been self-evident that living creatures were born only as male or female, and there was no need to think of a substance that might be responsible for this.

Only major deviations from this scheme could have aroused curiosity and perturbed this outlook, but such cases were extremely rare. Whenever an occasional child was born bisexual, there were priests at hand to relate how this was the gods' way of helping a nymph woo the son of Hermes and Aphrodite. One became accustomed to calling them hermaphrodites, even worshiped them as demigods—perhaps attracted by their magical aura—and then forgot the problem.

It was probably the natural logic with which the effects of the steroid hormones were built into the course of life that prevented man, well into modern times, from asking questions about the cause of his own identity. Life was as natural as the sky was high, the clouds were white and the leaves green. It was as natural as the fact that living creatures "naturally" had testes because they were male, or "naturally" had ovaries because they were female. No one asked the question the other way around: Was it possible that, perhaps, human beings only looked male because they had testes, or female because they had ovaries?

Farmers must have been among the first to have their doubts. Experience had taught them that removal of the testes of domestic animals not only caused sterility but initiated other changes as well. Cats became fat and good-natured, cocks lost their proud tail feathers, and ferocious bulls were turned into tame oxen. As far as the farmers were concerned, the primary reason for such operations was to bring about these changes.

However, if farmers had their doubts, we have no record of any. Even Aristotle, who described the consequences of caponization in great detail, apparently failed to penetrate to the logical conclusion that the removal of "something," with its consequences, meant the original presence of "something" else. In other words, in the normal cock, something must have existed which produced the handsome tail feathers to begin with.

Admittedly, any experiment performed by the methods of those times would not have supported such a theory, Bulls' testes were consumed out of the same magical desire as were the hearts of lions, but since testosterone is destroyed in the stomach, no effect was observed. However, when has lack of evidence ever hurt a theory? Had there not been philosophers prior to Copernicus who speculated that the earth revolves around the sun—without being able to prove it? No, lack of evidence was not the problem. The simple truth was that the individual had not yet met his Copernicus who could displace him from his central position. Man was as he was. It was up to the natural sciences of modern times to dethrone the *self* as the measure of all things in order to turn it into nothing more than a resultant of impersonal biosystems.

Nevertheless, lack of a theoretical concept did not prevent people in ancient and medieval times from studying and utilizing the consequences of expertly performed dehormonizations. Of special interest were the character changes noticed after accidental or deliberate castration, for instance in eunuchs. Even in those times, man was trying to transcend himself, to "expand his mind." It was inevitable that this quest would lead him to seek a way in which character change could be accomplished.

During Hellenistic times, the priests of Cybele practiced self-emasculation in order to be closer to the goddess. Jesus Christ (Matt. 19:12) spoke of "eunuchs who made themselves eunuchs for the sake of the kingdom of heaven," although he added, "He who is able to accept this, let him accept it." The possibility of character modification has always stirred man's imagination, and the Valerians of medieval times, as well as the Skoptze sect of modern Russia, looked upon self-mutilation as a religious duty.

This does not mean that the physical consequences of castration were overlooked. Abelard and the medieval castrato choirs reflect an accurate knowledge of the psysiology of sex hormones and their ability to maintain sexual function or to preserve a particular voice range. Yet it was always the details of removal which were studied while, strangely enough, there were still no questions asked about the possible existence of a substance determining the normal condition.

Modern times approached, and still the idea of a substance such as a hormone had not been conceived. Finally, in 1849, the physiologist Berthold of Göttingen drew the logical conclusion that it must also be possible to add something, if it is possible to remove something. During an experiment in which he implanted testicular tissue from mature cocks into young ones, he experienced, for the first time, the artificial maturation of a cock's comb. He described his sensational findings with classic simplicity.

"On August 2 of last year, I caponized six young cocks, namely a, b, c, three months, and d, e, f, two months old. None of these animals had its wattles, comb, or spurs removed. Both testes of cocks a and d were removed; these animals, later on, displayed entirely the nature of capons, behaved cowardly, rarely engaged in brief fights with other cocks, and exhibited the familiar monotonous capon voice. Comb and wattles turned pale and showed little development; the head remained small. When these animals were killed on December 20, there was an insignificant, barely noticeable scar where the testes had been. The spermatic ducts were thin, fragile little threads.

Cocks b and c were castrated in the same manner, however, only one testis was removed while the other one remained, isolated, in the abdominal cavity. On the other hand, cocks c and f had both testes removed from the abdominal cavity and then, one testis of cock c was placed into the abdominal cavity of cock f and one testis from cock f into the abdominal cavity of cock e, between the intestines.

In their general behavior, these four cocks (b, e, c, f) displayed the nature of uncastrated animals; they crowed quite soundly, often engaged in fights with each other and with other young cocks, and showed the usual inclination toward the hens; moreover, their combs and wattles developed as in ordinary cocks.

Berthold was not only a keen observer and experimenter, but also a logical thinker. He came to the conclusion (which was not exactly self-evident at the time) that implantation of the donor tissue alone could not be responsible for the effect. Rather, since there was no nervous connection, there must have been a substance which reached the feathers and comb through the circulatory system. Sterling later coined the term hormones (Greek: *horman* = to stir up) for those substances which, secreted by glands in small quantities, produce their effects in areas remote from their points of origin. Berthold concludes:

The peculiar consensual and antagonistic relationship between individual and social life which becomes particularly pronounced during puberty and lasts into old age, is not absent even with the testes removed from their original location as well as from their nerves, and healed to an entirely different part of the body. Judging by voice, reproductive drive, eagerness to fight, and growth of comb and wattles, such animals remain true cocks. However, transplanted testes can no longer have connections with their original nerves and, as becomes clear from the third sentence, there are no specific nerves governing secretion. Therefore it follows that the consensus in question is determined by the productive condition of the testes, i.e. by their effect on the blood and

> then by the corresponding effect of the blood on the general organism of which, it is true, the nervous system is a very essential part."

At that time, those were revolutionary words.

During the same year, a Scottish physician, Thomas Addison, discovered a relationship between the adrenal glands and the bronzed-skin disease which was subsequently named after him and about which we will report at a later point. Could it be possible that Berthold's method held the key to a future cure for this deadly disease?

The fire of enthusiasm was spreading and the dream of everlasting youth became an obsession. The concept of nervous regulation of all life processes, which had prevailed in medicine since Descartes without yielding any tangible results, was discarded with relief in favor of secretory control. In 1855, Claude Bernard publicized the function of the liver as a gland, and his compatriot Brown-Séquard experimentally confirmed Addison's findings of a connection between the bronzed-skin disease and the adrenal glands. However, the official beginning of the hormone era was June 1, 1889, when Brown-Séquard, then 72 years old, presented himself to an amazed college of physicians as the rejuvenated product of a testicular extract treatment. For a while, some of his adversaries may have passed sarcastic remarks about his rejuvenation being so thorough that the old man immediately came down with whooping cough, but the concept of a chemical messenger, giving orders to the tissues as to when and how to grow, prevailed. At this historic moment, a steroid hormone was put on the same level with the bile acids, cholesterol and the cardiac glycosides. From then on, hormones were considered as true substances.

Still missing was the realization that both rickets, which afflicted the children of miners, and the pupation of insects were initiated by similar substances. Nevertheless, the first steps had been taken. The actual existence of a hormone, however, remained to be demonstrated; the active substance remained to be isolated. Up to now, removal and/or implantation of tissue had permitted an indirect conclusion about such a substance, but no one could point to an individual crystal and say, "This is the substance that causes the change." Nor was it possible to recognize, based on elucidation of the chemical structure, that these all belonged to the same group of substances, for the generic term "steroids" had not yet been coined.

In addition, a peculiar dilemma existed. The amounts of hormones secreted in the human or animal body are so inconceivably small that they could

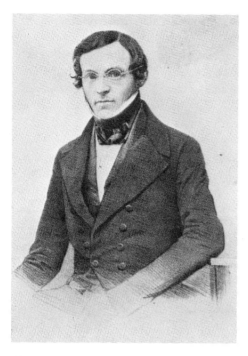

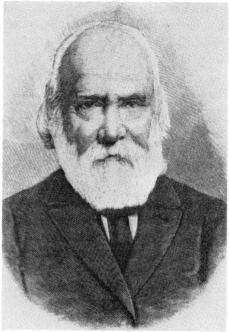

Fig. 2-1. Arnold Adolph Berthold, 1803–1861.

Fig. 2-2. Charles Edouard Brown-Séquard, 1817–1894.

only be discovered with the help of a steroid chemistry elaborated in the most minute detail. Chemists, however, had no reason for developing this kind of chemistry since they had no inkling that it would lead to the discovery of hormones. On the other hand, hormone researchers, not realizing that they were working with steroids, might just as well have asked for help from protein chemistry or any of the other thousands of specialized branches, which would, of course, have proved futile. Therefore, it had to be left to chance whether steroid chemistry would receive enough impetus from other directions so that, one day, it would cross the path of the hormone researchers. This lucky coincidence took place in early nineteenth-century Paris.

There, while Napoleon was marching across Europe, a 26-year-old chemist by the name of Michel Chevreul, had been pondering what chemical mysteries of the world awaited his discovery. He proceeded to win fame as the first to recognize a relationship between the colors of chemical compounds and their structures, and must have been an ironic character who, although advanced in years, still wrote a paper which he entitled "Diversion of a Member of the

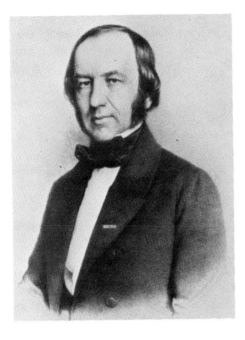

Fig. 2-3. Claude Bernard, 1813–1878.

Institute of France while the King of Prussia, William I, Was Laying Siege to Paris." In 1812, he began to occupy himself with the investigation of fats which, when combined with caustic soda, usually turn into soaps. Then, one day, he came upon a puzzling group of fats, none of which would turn into soap when combined with caustics. He called them "nonsaponifiable fats." Among the fats which surprised him in this manner, was the one that could be recovered from gallstones. Since the word gall is derived from the Greek *chole* and since, furthermore, this strange "fat" remained solid (*stereos*) even at a temperature of 100°C, he named it cholesterol. However, since neither he nor other scientists found this discovery very exciting, it was put on the shelf. Little did they know what they were missing.

In the mid-nineteenth century, a Heidelberg physiologist, Gmelin, who studied diseases of the liver, succeeded in isolating from bile an additional substance which he recognized as the therapeutically active component of the traditional *fel tauri desiccata,* dried ox bile. Since it reacted as an acid, Gmelin named it "bile acid." However, other than the fact that both substances were present in bile, there appeared to be no connection.

Several years later, the French set out to isolate the cardiac-active components of the purple foxglove and other plants, as well as those of the African arrow poisons, without any knowledge of their structure. Subsequently,

Charles Tanret discovered an additional nonsaponifiable fat, this time of vegetable origin, in yeast fungi. For the first time, he disclosed a molecular formula for one of these nonsaponifiable substances. Boldly he asserted that each molecule of his "ergosterol" consisted of exactly 28 carbon atoms, 44 hydrogen atoms and only a single oxygen atom. Anyone was free to go ahead and check his count! It took 30 years until someone did—and verified the analysis.

Similar molecular formulas for the bile acids and the digitalis poisons suggested that they were somehow related, which was later confirmed by Wieland. And that was the end of it. The hormones stubbornly resisted discovery.

To some chemically oriented demigod watching over developments, it might have seemed, even as late as the turn of the century, that the two would never meet: steroid chemistry, listlessly plodding along its desolate, arid road, and hormone physiology on its hectic, ever frustrating course. However, events would soon prove this mere demigod wrong.

Even then there were men who doggedly pursued steroid chemistry for reasons unknown to themselves, while other men continuously invented new ways of isolating hormonal substances. These were no longer mere dilettantes or amateurs, but dedicated scientists who would never have solved this problem without devoting their lives to it completely. Such men were eventually destined to meet, regardless of their starting point.

3. Discovering the Mountains Below

The Discovery of the Biological Steroids and their Target Areas in the Process of Life

CHOLESTEROL AND THE CELL MEMBRANE

To understand steroids, it is necessary to understand cholesterol. The chemical determination of cholesterol is child's play. One needs only to get a hold of a gallstone, scrape off a few crystals, dissolve them in chloroform, and shake them in sulfuric acid. A beautiful, deep-red coloration, slowly turning purple, indicates the presence of cholesterol. Cholesterol is everywhere. The human body contains about 300 grams (g). It is present in especially high concentration in the brain and in egg yolk, but it also occurs in the arteries of arteriosclerotics. This is where it first became clinically significant, at the same time providing a stimulus to steroid research. However, these shiny yellow patches which obstruct the most important blood vessels or impair their elasticity, and kill one-third of all human beings while turning others into cerebral sclerotics, gave no clues as to the function of cholesterol. They are nothing but a wrong turn in the metabolic process, which will be discussed at a later point. The real significance of cholesterol is more fundamental.

Cholesterol is the substance chosen by all animal cells to render their membranes selectively permeable. This involves both the shape and the distribution of electrical charges, which we need not go into. Because of its special molecular properties, cholesterol allows certain important substances to pass through the cell membrane, while barring others, thus enabling the cell to differentiate not only between different substances but also between "inside" and "outside." For the cell membrane, this semiliquid marvel, containing but a few molecules, must have some "intelligence" which enables it to let waste materials pass from the cell to its environment, and prevent noxious substances from getting in and life-sustaining materials from getting out. It is the function of cholesterol to endow the cell with this kind of intelligence. This is accomplished by means of its electrical and fat- or water-repellent properties, respectively. Obviously, cholesterol is one of the most important components of the membrane; and although we still know far too little about the function of this small, flat disc, we already have a fairly good idea of its position relative to the other membrane molecules (see Fig. 3-1). Furthermore, cholesterol is the parent substance of all animal steroids including the steroid hormones.

It took a long time for cholesterol to reveal its secrets. After Chevreul described it in 1812, a hundred years went by without its yielding any additional information. Finally, around the turn of the century, a new chemistry set out to examine this substance—a chemistry that pursued the envisioned goal systematically and purposefully until it was attained. Its disciples were professional scientists who had rolled up their sleeves. Steroids had always been the research domain of the young. Chevreul was 26 when he discovered them as a separate class of substances, and again, it was a young chemist who, in 1913, took the second big step in the investigation of the steroids: elucidation of their structure.

The man whose life's goal it was to reveal the nature of cholesterol and the steroids was just 27 years old when he made up his mind. He was Adolf Windaus, the son of a textile manufacturer. Originally, it had been his parents' wish that he take over his father's mill.

But this was the era of discoveries; Louis Pasteur and Robert Koch had captured the hearts of the young, and Windaus decided to study medicine. In the course of his studies, he attended lectures by the great chemist Emil Fischer, under whose influence he eventually turned to chemistry.

At age 36, Windaus received a professorship at Innsbruck and, two years later, he was called to Göttingen as professor ordinarius, where he quickly won international recognition as the foremost expert on steroids. Why he chose to study steroids is difficult to determine. Butenandt, who knew him very well, believes that Windaus felt instinctively, almost in a flash of genius, that he was dealing with something of great importance. This was certainly quite remarkable, especially in view of the fact that, at the time, the substances called steroids were not really very interesting: a few secretory products of the gall bladder, the poison from a plant, the fat-like extract of ergot, some foam-producing saponins.

Windaus' first problem was to establish definitively what substances actually belonged to the category of steroids. He needed a quick and sure means for identifying and isolating them. Fortunately, he came upon a publication asserting that cholesterol destroys the powerful toxic effect of

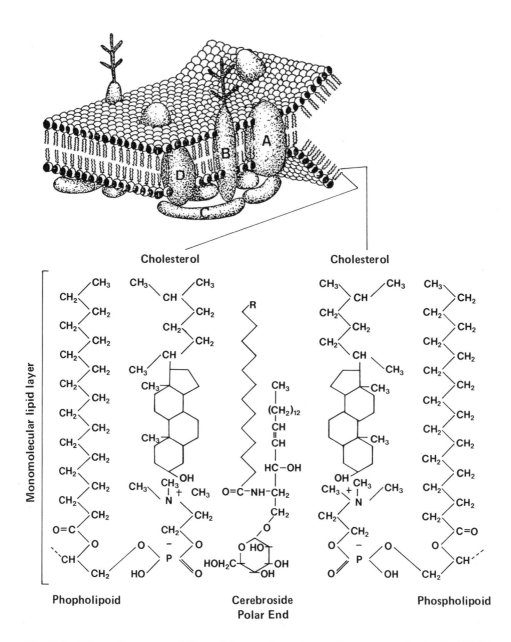

Fig. 3-1. Schematic representation of the erythrocyte membrane according to the "fluid mosaic" model.

digitonin on red blood corpuscles. From this he concluded that such detoxification resulted from a precipitate formed by cholesterol in combination
with the toxic digitonin (Fig. 3-2), and he assumed that other steroids would
likewise form precipitates with digitonin—thus allowing them to be recognized and isolated from solutions. It turned out that he was right.

Following this methodological success, he spent the next 20 years creating
some order among the many steroids which, thanks to his new method, were
suddenly being discovered by researchers everywhere. Any other scientist
might have been sidetracked by this multitude of new compounds, but
although Windaus worked conscientiously with many different kinds of
steroids, he always returned to cholesterol. This substance continued to be
his main interest.

In this manner, Windaus worked for over 20 years and, for some time, no
one attributed any significance to his results. If his work has made him
the father of steroid chemistry, a considerable portion of his success
must be credited to his personality. Windaus pursued his goal with a mono-
mania that belied his otherwise liberal and worldly nature. One would have
liked to be there, when he moved from group to group among his students,

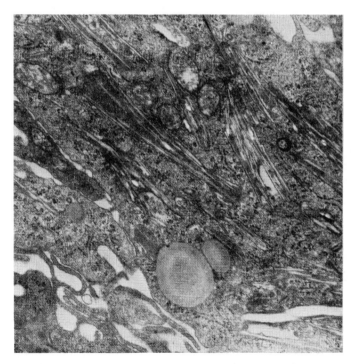

Fig. 3-2. Crystals of cholesterol digitonide in a macrophage cell (electron microscope).

reserved yet friendly, hands clasped behind his back, rarely praising, silence his only mode of disapproval. This is how Butenandt describes him:

> His speech was concise and to the point, he loathed small talk and appeared to have no use for poetical quotations. At the Institute, he radiated a serenity that greatly encouraged our work and nipped in the bud each loud word, each unprofessional argument. His sense of justice and veracity placed Windaus into dangerous opposition to the Nazi rulers to whom he refused to make any concessions. His candor and his courage, his personal integrity in facing the period from 1933 to 1945, dulled the weapons of those who repeatedly tried to discredit him or his institute.

By 1926, Windaus' research in the chemistry of cholesterol (and many other steroids) had advanced to a point where the only thing still missing was the final structural formula. He was not to succeed in determining this until 1932. However, before this dream came true, he was to be confronted with another steroid.

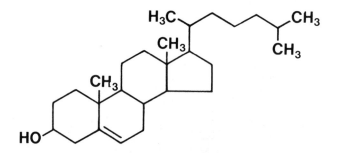

Fig. 3-3. Structural formula of cholesterol.

Windaus' fame had spread in the scientific community, and from all parts of the world, students came to Göttingen. The assistants who worked for him, sometimes as many as 200, carried the incredible story of his accomplishments and his humanity back to their own countries. One day, from one of those countries, came the first reaction that was to confirm Windaus' intuitive recognition of the importance of this group of substances.

VITAMIN D AND THE SKELETAL FRAMEWORK

Finding information about rickets in a modern medical textbook is not easy. This disfiguring and often fatal disease, which had plagued Europe since the times of Neanderthal man, has practically disappeared. It is true that we occasionally still see some of its victims from the period prior to 1920: elderly people, their bones depleted of calcium by the disease, hunchbacked or bowlegged, or afflicted with deformities of skull and chest. However, with few exceptions, rickets no longer affects Europe.

Many years ago, people on the European continent had been able, thanks to the Gulf Stream, to settle in northern latitudes which were uninhabitable in Siberia and Alaska, but they had paid the price: rickets. The Neanderthal people had not been spared, and the ancient Greeks with their keen eyes for clinical observation had used the word rachitis to denote a syndrome comprising all the various symptoms of rickets. Around 1650, rickets unexpectedly increased in intensity. Starting in England, and therefore known as the English disease, it swept across Europe along with the smog of industrialization. There were many theories about its causes, but the real reason was not known. Yet, the answer was clearly there, in the descriptions of the disease, but no one knew how to read between the lines.

In the early nineteenth century, G. Wendelstadt, in his description of the "diseases of Wetzlar" told of the swollen limbs and enlarged heads of the children, just sitting there waiting for death, in their homes huddled along dark and narrow alleys. Only what was the reason for this? Was it Wetzlar, itself, or its industrial character?

Meanwhile, in England, which had much experience in this respect, people were puzzling over the fact that no cases of rickets occurred in rural areas, while in London and Manchester, rich and poor alike were stricken with the disease—even the lions in the zoo. Also, people who lived in Dublin stayed healthy. Perhaps a geographical factor was involved—something in the soil of Wetzlar or London?

In Germany, Kassowitz drew attention to another variable: the season of the year. He noticed a greater frequency of new cases during the winter months. Hansemann confirmed that most children who were born in the fall and died in the following spring had been suffering from rickets, while those who were born in the spring and died in the fall, had been spared this disease.

To complicate matters further, others observed that European children could be cured of rickets on the island of Java. Could it be the difference in diet? However, missionaries to Japan and Manchuria reported that rickets was unknown in these countries even though nutrition was rather poor. Perhaps it was a racial peculiarity of the Europeans after all?

It was the brilliant missionary Theobald Palm who, in 1890, reading a detailed description of the living conditions of children in faraway countries, identified the common factor that had been overlooked by all other observers: the lack of sunlight in the lives of the rachitic children and the sunny climate where the children were healthy!

All of a sudden, the other reports began to make sense: It had been the smog above London and Manchester, blocking the sunlight, that had mimicked a geographical distribution, and it had been the winter sun, low on the horizon, that had been responsible for the seasonal distribution noted by Kassowitz.

Nevertheless, to begin with, this was only a theory. It took 22 years until it could be proved by an animal experiment. In 1912, in Paris, Jan Raczynski raised two newborn puppies under exactly the same conditions, with one exception—one of them was kept away from sunlight. After six weeks, the shade-dog developed rickets, while its sun-sibling stayed healthy. Palm's sun theory had been verified.

A wave of clinical testing began, first of all in those countries where there was plenty of sunshine. It was found that in India, despite the sun, there were rachitic children in rich families who kept their children in "purdah," i.e., in the dark, secluded quarters of the house. Taking those children outside, into the sunlight, immediately confirmed its miraculous effect. This was easy to do in India, but how could Europeans provide enough light when the winter sun never rises more than 30° above the horizon? They built large, glass enclosures to allow rachitic patients to remain outdoors in the winter, but these early attempts at therapy failed because things were not as simple as initially assumed. It was not yet known that the window panes of these so-called solaria rather efficiently blocked the therapeutically effective ultraviolet component of light. Instead, it was believed that the radiation intensity was simply too low. Consequently, in Germany, Buchholz built solaria with high-intensity carbon filament lamps, but his tests were not successful either. Then, in 1919, Berlin pediatrician Huldschinsky tried quartz-lamp radiation treatments on four children and cured them of rickets within two months. Huldschinsky's discovery finally revealed that it was the invisible waves of the solar spectrum (290–320 nm) that effectively cured rickets.

Yet it was still not known how this occurred. Again, it was Huldschinsky who performed an ingenious experiment. He irradiated only one arm of a rachitic child with quartz light and then proved by means of X-rays that the other arm had been restored to health as well. Thus, it was established that light had no direct influence on the bone, but that it helped the body form a substance which was distributed through the blood. Did this mean that a hormone was involved?

A conjecture of this sort could not go uncontested for, at the same time, there were scientists who refused to give up the idea that rickets might be caused by some *nutritional* factor. (To distinguish them from the advocates of the sun theory, they were known as the "London school.") Their approach was supported by the observation that it was possible to induce rickets in experimental animals through a diet that was low in phosphates (or rich in butter). They argued that if sunlight was so important, why did Eskimos not have rickets when they spent six months of the year in polar darkness? Perhaps a vitamin really was the important factor?

Such an explanation was by no means absurd. This was the time when vitamins were coming into use. What could seem more natural than to assume that rickets was likewise caused by a vitamin deficiency? Nutritional experiments with rats showed that certain oily foods were indeed therapeutically effective. This brought to mind the diet of the Eskimos and spawned the idea of using cod-liver oil. In 1917, Hess proved the remedial quality of cod-liver oil administered to rachitic negro children in New York. Instead of expensive sun-lamp treatments, it was sufficient to take a spoonful of cod-liver oil each day! Rickets was no longer a problem.

However, the question remained: Was the substance involved a hormone or a vitamin? Was it something produced in the body, or something essential that had to be provided by external sources? Two diametrically opposed hypotheses confronted each other. Again, it was Hess who had the brilliant idea to reconcile the two. Was it not conceivable, he thought, that ultraviolet radiation does nothing more than act on the skin, converting a previously consumed provitamin into the same substance that was the active ingredient of cod-liver oil? In that case, then, could ultraviolet radiation perhaps produce the same effect outside the body? Without further ado, Hess, and later Steenbock, irradiated rat feed which, it was hoped, contained the necessary provitamin. Working independently, they both discovered (as happens so often when the time is ripe) that irradiated feed produced antirachitic effects in these animals. The vitamin theory had won, for the time being.

Immediately, scientists set about isolating either the vitamin or the provitamin. It was called vitamin D, but that was not really of any help. One, two, three years elapsed while scientists irradiated, distilled, filtrated, and extracted, but they did not find the vitamin, or the provitamin, in cod-liver oil. It was able to slip through the dragnet of modern chemistry which, at the time, could detect and isolate even milligram amounts of substances. At one point, researchers confused the wanted substance with vitamin A, which was incidentally discovered this way, but once the error was cleared up, they were once more running in place. Never had chemistry encountered such a striking failure, except in the search for the likewise hypothetical sex hormones, a fact that was neither helpful nor generally noticed.

It soon became obvious that both vitamin D and the elusive provitamin had to be fats (rather than proteins or carbohydrates) and that they were not to be found among the oils proper but, surprisingly, among the baffling group of nonsaponifiable fats which, years ago, had been shelved as insignificant by Chevreul. However, these peculiar substances, which constituted tiny traces of "contaminants" in oils, were virgin territory as far as chemistry was concerned. Their structure was not known, nor were the means available for separating them successfully and testing them for vitamin D activity.

After lengthy investigation, scientists focused their efforts on two of the steroids (as we call them today), animal cholesterol and vegetable ergosterol, both of which are present in trace amounts in cod-liver oil. However, due to the yet imperfect methods of separation, these two steroids initially still contained trace amounts of impurities. Then something strange happened: the more one succeeded in removing these contaminants, the lower the vitamin D activity became.

Suddenly, it became clear that scientists had been following the wrong road. The steering wheel had to be turned 180°. Instead of continuing their work on cholesterol and ergosterol, researchers pounced upon the "impurities" in them. Could they be the sought-for vitamin D? Difficulties encountered in separating them from the aforementioned steroids were indications of a very close chemical relationship. However, this too proved to be a disappointment. The impurity turned out to be yet another complex of unknown substances with varied vitamin D activity, which resisted further separation by the methods then available. Nevertheless, in the course of these events, one thing had become certain—the hypothetical vitamin and its provitamin had to be steroids. As soon as the problem had been narrowed down to the search for an unknown steroid, Hess decided in 1926 to ask for help from Windaus, then the "greatest expert on sterols." For the first time, applied therapeutical research could not continue without the Göttingen group and its expertise. "The lonesome road of sterol chemistry," as Butenandt once called it, had come to an end. Physiology and chemistry had met at last. (Fig. 3–4.)

Hess and Windaus started out by identifying the cholesterol impurities. They discovered that there were countless variants, any one of them potentially antirachitic, differing only in the location of a hydrogen atom or a double bond. Testing all of them for vitamin D activity turned out to be an enormously time-consuming project; the separation of these substances, which were barely distinguishable chemically, required exquisite sensitivity and superhuman patience. Each time painstaking labor finally yielded a new cholesterol fraction, it had to be irradiated and then tested for vitamin D activity. For this purpose, it was necessary to induce experimental rickets in rats and subsequently inject the animals with the material to be tested. Then three to four weeks were required for the results to be conclusive. However, the outcome was always negative. After Windaus and his assistants had completed this tedious testing program with 30 different cholesterol derivatives, they finally turned their attention to the ergosterol group.

Meanwhile, the Göttengen physicist Pohl had invented an optical method which made it possible to determine, within three or four hours, the presence of activatable material by observing the mysterious processes that take place during conversion of the provitamin to vitamin D. By this method, it was soon found that a certain impurity of the ergosterol group indeed contained the desired provitamin.

Initially, there were high hopes that the problem might be solved, but additional testing once again cast the shadow of disappointment on these results. The suspected ergosterol impurity, traceable only in minute amounts, turned out to be nothing but another confusing complex of many elusive steroids consisting of oxidation products, isomers, and reduction products, whose existence had been hitherto unknown. It was like fighting the many-headed Hydra—each head, when cut off, was replaced by seven others. It soon became obvious that the ergosterol structure would have to be elucidated before any further progress was possible.

At this crucial point, development was halted for some time by Windaus' belief in fair play. Several years earlier, he had granted a request from Reindel in Munich, to place him in charge of investigating the structure of

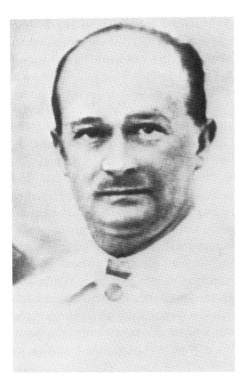

Fig. 3-4. Adolf Windaus, 1876-1959.

ergosterol. Now that the importance of its structure in the search for vitamin D had suddenly become obvious, Windaus refused to take the project away from Reindel who was working desperately, assisted by only a few students. Windaus found himself at the threshold of an extremely important discovery, perhaps the culmination of his life's work, yet it was more important to him to keep his word. Even he, however, could not continue for very long to control the progress of world-wide research. Once the importance of ergosterol became known, investigators went to work feverishly to find out which of its derivatives was converted into vitamin D on irradiation. Reluctantly, Windaus succumbed to the pressure for results on the part of the Medical Research Institute in London and his student Linsert in Elberfeld. He authorized work on the structure of ergosterol and, four years later, isolated a highly antirachitic product which he initially named vitamin D_1. This designation already indicated that he expected to discover additional vitamins. Simultaneously, the English found a similarly active preparation which they called calciferol.

Very soon, both Windaus and the British realized that, once again, they had isolated a complex, this time of pure vitamin D and an inactive constituent, lumisterol. However, it now took only a short time to isolate the pure vitamin D, named vitamin D_2 by Windaus and calciferol-new by the British. It was an ergosterol derivative in which ring B of the molecule had opened. (For a long time it was believed that ergosterol is the direct precursor of vitamin D. It was not until many years later that the Frenchman Velluz was able to establish the structure of the actual provitamin, so that, to this day, ergosterol is still called the provitamin.)

Vitamin D_2 is a highly potent substance. To prevent rickets, it is sufficient to ingest .01 milligram (mg) of this vitamin daily. In comparison to the previous tablespoonful of cod-liver oil, the potency had been successfully increased by a factor of one million. For the first time, it was possible to reach this low order of magnitude with a "vitamin." This, and the fact that none of the other vitamins was a steroid, should have been food for thought, but, for the time being, one was satisfied to know that irradiation of ergosterol, in food or in the skin, would yield the life-saving vitamin.

One or two things were still a mystery, however. For example, where did the body's vitamin D normally originate? It was certain that the average human diet, with the exception of fish, scarcely contained any vitamin D_2. If it appeared strange that the essential vitamin as such was not present in our food, it was even more peculiar that the provitamin, which is converted to vitamin D in the skin by irradiation, was a *vegetable* steroid that the body could neither synthesize nor obtain from food in guaranteed sufficient amounts. Therefore, it remained unclear why the human organism, capable of synthesizing so many steroids, should be dependent upon vegetable sources for this most vital steroid. Nevertheless, the ergosterol content of foods continued to be the indicator of their antirachitic quality.

Then, in 1934, a man by the name of Wedell noticed that, strangely enough, rickets in chickens could be cured by an amount of cod-liver oil that was less than indicated by its ergosterol fraction. Logically, this effect could only be due to the cholesterol fraction. A great deal of confusion resulted. After so many years of work, it suddenly seemed that an additional vitamin had been overlooked, one whose provitamin was probably derived from cholesterol after all and which was effective in even smaller amounts than vitamin D_2 –otherwise it could not have gone undetected at the time.

Again, work began at Göttingen. Windaus had, in the meantime, become famous. In 1928, he was awarded the Nobel Prize for his investigation of vitamin D. Yet he still chose to remain in the background–going from group to group in his unpretentious manner, stimulating research, assigning responsibility, and standing back whenever one of his collaborators discovered something important. Often, the acknowledgements in his students' papers were the only evidence of the role he actually played through his great experience and wise guidance.

Windaus must have realized at an early stage that his laboratory, with all its accumulated experience, would have no difficulty in finding this additional, even more potent, vitamin D. He renounced all claims to further honors and graciously left it to young Brockmann to take another look at the cholesterol fraction of cod-liver oil. Within the year, the mysterious provitamin was isolated: Mixed with the cholesterol were minute traces of 7-dehydrocholesterol which, on irradiation, afforded a new and even more potent vitamin D. It was named vitamin D_3. In chickens, vitamin D_3 was found to have 100 times the potency of vitamin D_2 (see Fig. 3–5).

At last, the riddle was solved. Our body *can* synthesize cholesterol and, therefore, its own provitamin D_3. This is deposited in the skin for irradiation and conversion to vitamin D_3. Consequently, the original hormone theory was restored to equal status with the vitamin theory. While vitamins are essential substances that must be supplied from external sources, hormones are, by definition, active substances which the organism itself is able to synthesize. This is the distinction between *vitamin* D_2 and *hormone* D_3.

What, one may ask, is the story of this strange hormone whose chain of production is interrupted at a crucial point where it cannot continue without sunlight? Was it always like this during the evolution of animals? Looking at animals that live in darkness, such as rats and certain deep-sea fish, we find that they can produce their vitamin D_3 from cholesterol *without* any help from the sun. Apparently, man has lost this ability. The step from 7-dehydro-

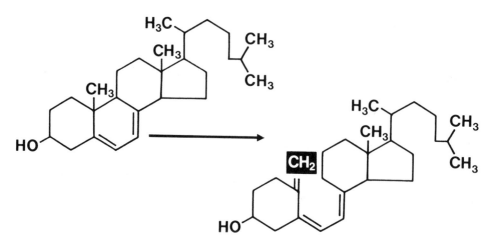

Fig. 3–5. 7-Dehydrocholesterol and vitamin D_3.

cholesterol to vitamin D_3 represents the weak link in the chain since, in the human organism, this conversion takes place in the skin and requires sun irradiation.

After this process, the steroid returns to the endocrine system deep within the body where it is converted to the actual hormone. According to the latest research findings, D_3 is still not the final active substance, but an intermediate product which travels from the skin to the liver where it receives an additional hydroxyl group at atom C-25, to become 25-hydroxy-cholecalciferol (25-HCC). Finally, in the kidney, another hydroxyl group (–OH) is added, this time to C-1. This hormone, 1,25-dihydroxycholecal-ciferol (or 1,25-DHCC), was found to be 10,000 times more potent than D_3 when tested in bone cultures.

Now that D_3 has been classified as a hormone, does it necessarily follow that D_2 is a vitamin? No, because if it is possible, whenever there is not enough light, to replace hormone D_3 with less potent vitamin D_2 from external sources, then D_2 can be categorized more accurately as a medication than an essential vitamin. Since vitamin D_2 is not needed when there is adequate sunlight, the situation is comparable to what happens with diabetes. The diabetic's injection of pig insulin—differently structured and somewhat less potent than the human variety—is clearly not an essential vitamin but rather a replacement for the missing hormone, i.e., a medication.

However, this is not necessarily always the case. Fish which live far from the sun, in the darkness of the ocean, probably receive their vitamin D_2 (passed on to us in fish-liver oil) directly or indirectly from plankton whose

7-dehydrocholesterol or ergosterol is subjected to sun irradiation on the ocean surface. For these fish, it would be a true vitamin, although it is now being claimed that some can make their own vitamin D.

One might ask what difference it makes whether D_3 is a vitamin or a hormone. To begin with, it means that the body needs vitamin D_2 only as a medicine, i.e., if something is wrong, and that it is therefore not necessary to administer it to everyone. It means, furthermore, that it is necessary to consider whether D_3, as a steroid hormone, may possibly be subject to the same rules and functions as the other steroid hormones which will be discussed in a subsequent chapter. The point is that vitamins are substances which represent parts of cell enzymes and simply do as they are told, while steroid hormones have intelligence. They are parts of a regulatory mechanism, with the steroid hormone playing a key role. The concept of vitamin D as a hormone has indeed led to the discovery of such a regulatory mechanism, which fulfills the vital function of maintaining blood calcium at a normal level.

Without going into complicated details, the following is a brief description of our present understanding of this regulatory mechanism and the role of vitamin D:

1. This particular mechanism operates to maintain blood calcium at a fixed level. This is important not only for the bones but also for many other body tissues.
2. A decrease in calcium level stimulates the parathyroid gland, an organ about the size of a cherry pit, adjacent but unrelated to the thyroid gland. The parathyroid gland then produces additional parathormone.
3. Parathormone stimulates the cortical substance of the kidney which converts the available supply of 25-HCC to 1,25-DHCC, i.e., the actual hormone D_3.
4. 1,25-DHCC activates transport of the necessary calcium through the intestinal wall into the blood stream and stimultaneously makes so-called amorphous calcium available from the bones.
5. As the calcium level rises, the production of parathormone, and, consequently, of the final stage of vitamin D is reduced. [Conversely, this mechanism can lower an excessive calcium level (see Fig. 3–6).]

Accordingly, this is a regulatory mechanism with so-called feedback similar to the control mechanisms we will find associated with all the steroid hormones, as discussed later in this text. Its components interact in such a manner that, even with fluctuations in consumption and supply, plasma

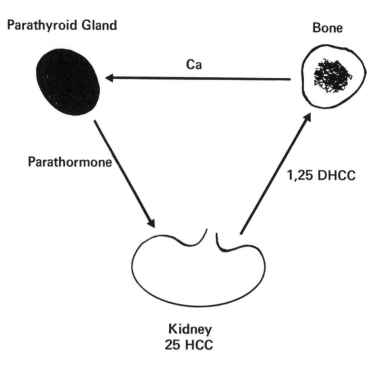

Fig. 3–6. Regulatory mechanism for vitamin D.

calcium always remains at the same normal level. The importance of this mechanism becomes obvious when we look at what happens if and when it malfunctions:

Hypercalcemia, i.e., excessive plasma calcium content, results in dangerous precipitation of calcium in certain tissues of the body, such as the kidneys, causing serious damage. This happens most frequently in cases of overdosage with vitamin D. An overdose of sun radiation is prevented by the fact that the identical wavelength (290–320 nm) which forms vitamin D in the skin, also produces a protective tan. From this point of view, the skin pigmentation of the negro can probably be understood as a protective mechanism against vitamin D poisoning.

In *hypocalcemia,* i.e., insufficient plasma calcium content, two different diseases may develop. A slow decrease in calcium level causes the dissolution of bone, a classic symptom of rickets. A rapid drop in blood calcium causes so-called tetanic spasms associated with a characteristic sharp flexion of the wrist joints. These spasms can be fatal without medical attention (a steroid, A.T.10, is used for therapy). Hypocalcemia develops under the following conditions:

1. Accidental removal of the parathyroid glands (e.g., during goiter surgery) leads to tetany due to the absence of parathormone.
2. Insufficient production of vitamin D in the skin leads to inadequate production of the hormone in the cortical substance of the kidney—and, consequently, to rickets—because of restricted availability of the raw material.
3. Failure (or removal) of the kidneys means loss of the endocrine gland normally activated by parathormone, and causes symptoms similar to rickets. This is one of the most serious secondary manifestations of certain kidney diseases in patients who could otherwise be kept alive for many years through dialysis and has only recently become fully understood.

Obviously, with modern research findings about the vitamin D mechanism, the original, naive conception of a "bone vitamin" has become rather shaky over the past few years. In fact, this problem, on which the books apparently had been closed some time ago, is once more a highly topical subject in clinical medicine, especially since there have been indications that a cure may soon be discovered for vitamin-D-refractory cases of rickets associated with diseases of the kidney.

This problem, in particular, has rekindled vitamin D research efforts, albeit without providing final answers to all the questions so far. As a matter of fact, additional questions have come up, for example, about the role of a recently discovered protein hormone, calcitonin, which is antagonistic to parathormone. Also, it has been established that certain other steroids can influence calcium metabolism, thus further complicating the picture. The female sex hormones act to retain calcium in the bone, whereas the corticoid hormones mobilize calcium and liberate it into the blood stream. This is a first intimation of a therapeutic problem we will encounter later on; in the effective spectra of the various steroids, there are areas of overlap which are responsible for so-called side-effects.

It is obvious that, after 50 years, the "problem of vitamin D" is far from settled. Even now, we still experience the ripples originating from a pebble that Windaus dropped into the water many years ago. However, nowadays we no longer erect monuments, except for those which bear witness to future generations of our greed and folly. Have we nothing else to communicate?

"When I try to imagine a monument to be erected, some day, out of humanity's gratitude for Windaus," said Wilhelm Biltz in 1941, "I see his figure surrounded by a crowd of children, cured and healthy thanks to him."

WIELAND'S FIRST STEROID FORMULA

Bile Acids and the Digestion of Fats

While all this was going on at Göttingen, there was another chemist, farther south, who, in contrast to the solitary, introverted Windaus, was continuously scanning all of chemistry for areas that might possibly interest him. Heinrich Wieland was a determined, unceremonious man with a natural sense of humor, the son of a chemist in Pforzheim, the heart of the German goldsmiths' art. While a young instructor, over a period of 20 years, he had explored anything in nature that appeared worth knowing, just so long as it contained nitrogen—morphine, curare, strychnine, the poison of the destroying angel mushroom. (Fig. 3–7.)

Then, suddenly, in 1912, he deviated from this practice and focused his attention on a group of substances that appeared rather dull and consisted of nothing but carbon, hydrogen, and a little oxygen—the *bile acids*. Why he did this, no one can say for sure. Possibly, it bothered him that very little

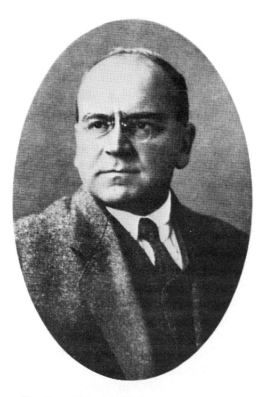

Fig. 3–7. Heinrich Wieland, 1877–1957.

was known about something that had been discovered such a long time ago. In addition, he may have been stimulated by the fact that success was still eluding Windaus after years of struggling with the related cholesterol and that the scientific community was beginning to take notice. Cheerfully, Wieland began his work.

However, this straightforward, clearheaded man of action—who would have preferred that all problems be solved immediately—had to come down a peg or two. Although he soon discovered that these substances had to have four interconnected rings, it took years before he and his assistants were able to break down those rings for detailed examination. This was attributable to the fact that Wieland, as well as Windaus, was working with chemistry's first carbon ring systems for which no methodology existed at the time.

Years went by, and Wieland was appointed professor ordinarius at Munich University, but success was nowhere in sight. This unexpected resistance ignited his fighting spirit. In 1828, Gmelin had first recovered impure cholic acid from ox bile; in 1848, Strecker had isolated the first pure bile acid; in 1885, a second bile acid was discovered and, in 1886, a third. Was it then to take another 50 years until the nature of these substances would finally be revealed?

Without neglecting his other work, but also without his usual quick results, Wieland spent year after year investigating the constitution of this peculiar substance called bile acid, fascinated by the discovery that it could change various substances from insoluble to water-soluble. One ring after another was explored, the work proceeding with such parallel concentration that Wieland, arriving at the lab in the morning, often asked half-jokingly, "Which ring are we working on today?" However, he remained patient. When the common features of cholesterol and the bile acids became increasingly evident, investigators at Munich and Göttingen were able to compare notes, and slowly came up with the tentative formula of a molecule that no one had ever seen (Fig. 3–8). At Munich, they were not too happy with this formula, but the world at large had gotten wind of the significance of these

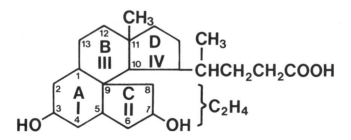

Fig. 3–8. First formula of desoxycholic acid (Wieland, 1928).

substances and, in 1927, Wieland was awarded the Nobel Prize for his work with "the bile acids and related substances."

Wieland's Nobel lecture reflects a memory of the ascetic years when he talks about a "long and unspeakably wearisome trek through the arid desert of structure"—whose end was nowhere in sight even then. However, at the same time, he intimates that these might be more than ordinary natural substances. He speaks of the magnitude of the problem, which strengthened his perserverance, and of his determination to explore the biological relationships within a field of related natural substances which "in addition to the bile acids, includes the sterols, and very likely also the vegetable cardiac poisons, the poisons from the skin secretions of toads and probably also other important substances such as certain vitamins." The term "important substances" makes it sound as though Wieland already had a premonition of the importance of the steroidal molecule and of the discoveries that, within a few years, were to follow one another in rapid succession, because he and Windaus had laid the foundations for the methodology.

Five more years were required, however, for the structural model of 1928, whose "unsightly corner at C-8" had irritated Butenandt's esthetic sense at the time, to achieve its final form. In 1932, after 20 years of incredibly tedious work, the decisive step forward suddenly came from two directions. Based on X-ray crystallographic analysis of steroids, a method developed by the English physicist Bernal, Rosenheim and King proposed the formula shown in Fig 3-9. Later that same year, Wieland and Dane modified this formula to the famous final version (Fig. 3-10). The first correct steroid formula had been discovered.

Wieland's name will come up again in our discussion of the toad poisons whose exploration he pioneered. In addition, he investigated the sterols of yeast and the hormones present in urine. Yet after he had solved the most difficult problem, his roving spirit was still more powerfully attracted to new

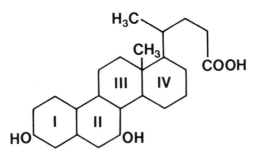

Fig. 3-9. Intermediate version of the first steroid formula by Rosenheim and King (May, 1932).

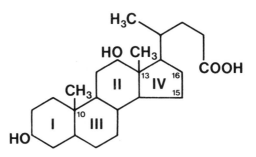

Fig. 3-10. Final version of the first steroid formula by Wieland and Dane (September, 1932), and Rosenheim and King (November, 1932).

areas of inquiry. He discovered a new group of chemical substances in the pigment of the brimstone butterfly which, during the rule of the Third Reich, earned him the reputation of an unrealistic dreamer. No one was aware, at the time, that the vital folic acid would, someday, be found to belong to this group. Most importantly, he elucidated the oxidation processes in the living cell. However, as far as steroid chemists are concerned, he will always be "bile acid Wieland."

What exactly is the importance of the bile acids to man, apart from the fact that they helped establish the structure of the steroids? We have already learned, in the case of vitamin D, that steroids are effective in milligram amounts, and we will find this to be true, even more so, for the steroid hormones. What, then, is the function of the 6 g of bile acid secreted by the human gall bladder each day? What is it that forces the human organism to use this phylogenetically ancient steroid, the only steroid with ring A still projecting downward and, therefore, as we will learn later on, not suitable as a hormone?

Obviously, the bile acids are somehow involved in the digestive process. But how? We remember Wieland's discovery that the bile acids, and in particular their salts, act on insoluble substances to render them water-soluble. We know that nutrients can be absorbed through the intestinal lining only if they are soluble. Fats in particular, the greatest energy suppliers per gram, have a problem being absorbed. A globule of oil weighing, say, 1 g, has no chance of passing through the cell membranes or the fine pores of the intestinal lining. To make this possible, fat must first be broken down into its constituents, glycerol and fatty acids, by the protein enzymes of the intestinal juice. However, in order to break down the fat, the enzymes must be able to make contact—their efficacy is dependent upon the amount of surface area they can reach. In the case of the fat globule, this area would be about 5 square centimeters (cm^2). No matter how large an amount of enzyme is available, it must wait until the topmost layer, .001 millimeter (mm) thick, of this 5 cm² surface has been partially digested and removed—a process that could take several days.

Here is where the bile acids perform their *first* important function. With their molecules fat-soluble at one end and water-soluble at the other, the fat-soluble ends hang on to the fat globule, while the intestinal juice pulls the water-soluble tails and, presto, the large globule is fragmented into minute particles called micelle. To what advantage? The fat surface exposed to enzyme action, initially 5 cm², has now grown to 1500 square meters (m²) through this process of emulsification—in other words, from the size of a postage stamp to the area of six tennis courts!

As a *second* function, the bile acids then activate the enzymes so that these can be even more effective in breaking down the fat into glycerol and fatty acids.

However, we now encounter another difficulty. Glycerol can be absorbed through the intestinal lining, but the three fatty acids, which are insoluble in water, cannot. So again, for the *third time,* the bile acids come to the rescue. They enclose the individual fatty acid molecule in a sandwich, their water-soluble ends facing out. In this combination, the entire unit can pass through the intestinal membrane. This reminds us of slices of bread which make the piece of ham between them easier on the stomach. (Fig. 3–11.)

Once absorbed into the lymph channels of the intestine, the sandwich disintegrates; the fatty acids recombine with their glycerol into fat which is conveyed to the bloodstream in the lymph (this appears milky white because of the absorbed fat). Then the bile acids return to the liver and, finally, to the gall bladder, and the cycle begins again. In this manner, a liter of bile each day helps digest the fats in our diet.

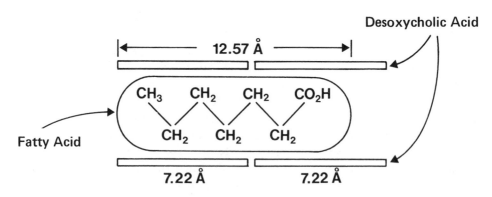

Fig. 3–11. "Fatty acid sandwich" (according to Fieser). For diffusion through the intestinal membrane, the bile acids enclose a fatty acid.

SEX HORMONES AND REPRODUCTION

The most magnificent moment in a bullfight is not the thrusting of the banderillas or the cuarto de la muerte. Instead, the most magnificent instant occurs when the bull trots into the arena and stops short, blinded by the sun. Five thousand aficionados hold their breath, staring at the black bull hesitantly pawing the sand. There is no sound but a child's soft crying. From the direction of the setting sun, a cool gust of wind sweeps across the square. The matador can sense the woman's eyes on him. Without looking, he adjusts his hat and squares his shoulders. Then, with carefully measured steps, he advances toward the bull.

This moment is so splendid because it is so full of meaning, full of strength and beauty. Male and female principle—*vive la différence!* There are few people who are aware of what lies behind all this—behind the 1200 pounds of concentrated strength and the gesture of the bullfighter; behind the woman, her jet-black hair spilling from her mantilla.

Giving the matter some thought, one might come up with the idea of hormones. However, to what extent are hormones actually involved? The answer is a long story—the story of *la différence.* It began about 300 million B.C. A few worms, snails and rare fish have survived from those times, and give us an inkling of what life was like without that difference which was to add so much verve and brilliance to the world; so much pain, yet so much love.

In those times, animals were hermaphrodites who lived life as best they could under such cheerless conditions. At most, they took an interest in the food supply and the rainfall, or possibly even paid some attention to outside temperatures. Meanwhile, somewhere in the brain, there sat an appendage, the hypophysis, which kept track of all this information. Whenever the season of the year, the spawning ground, and a few other variables seemed just right, the hypophysis dispatched tiny traces of two *protein hormones,* gonadotropins, to mobilize the primordial germ cells of these animals. When the germ cells had been discharged into the surrounding water or earth, and perhaps fertilized, and perhaps not eaten by their parents, then they perhaps developed into a new animal—an animal whose existence depended on coincidence. Too many "perhapses" restricted the phylogenetic development.

As evolution progressed, the requirements of the fertilized egg cell became more particular. A differentiated embryo needed improved protection and nourishment while growing. Moreover, each individual required more selective access to foreign genetic material in order to be able to develop into new life forms. Consequently, nature invented *sexual differentiation,* the separation of male and female principles, lying dormant in the hermaphrodite. Now, each party could specialize—the male to provide protection and the female to nurture the offspring. This involved tremendous transformations. The difficult task assigned by evolution to those animals that wanted to advance their development required three phases. The first necessitated physical *separation* of the potential male and female characteristics present in each individual, in order to accentuate them. In the second phase, the previously separated male and female were *reunited* for the purpose of mating; this was required in the service of evolution to accomplish fertilization. Finally, *synthesis* of the female and male principles, in a manner that would best serve for rearing the young, constituted the third phase, in which the mother would care for the young, and the father protect and feed them.

This was a tall order which the gonadotropins were unable to handle, since their previous function had been limited to stimulation of germ cell maturation by order from the brain. To accomplish these tremendous changes within the body, help was needed from substances which could induce the previously neutral body cells to *change* their preprogrammed goals in favor of the new tasks. This could be accomplished only by means of relatively complicated, flat molecules which, today, we call *steroid hormones.* These were available in large numbers to those primitive creatures and, from among them, nature selected two groups which had previous related experience: Controlled by the gonadotropins, these hormones had prepared the primitive gonoduct systems (the so-called Wolffian and Müllerian ducts, respectively) for passage of the germ cells, and they helped to support germ cell maturation. The group which was to effect masculinization is now called *androgenic;* the one which was to bring about feminization is called *estrogenic* (see Fig. 3–12). Because of their function, these two groups became known as the sex hormones. However, we must keep in mind that, despite this name, they had no direct connection with the ovum or the sperm.

The difficult trick, to begin with, was to effect the *separation* of the male and female in the first phase, i.e., to manipulate the fertilized, neutral ovum in such a way that it could develop into diametrical opposites. Initially, all fertilized ova possess the potential for later development of either male or female characteristics, and thus have the capacity to produce both male and female hormones at the same time. The consequent equilibrium of androgens and estrogens could not create the dynamic field, the polarity, which marks the course of our present lives. Therefore it was necessary, first of all, to create an imbalance—not only of steroids, but also of organs on which they would act, since each hormone needs its own specific target organ. Yet, how was this to be achieved?

The solution that nature came up with was brilliant. She decided to use the chromosomes for the purpose of creating two different sexes. We remember the chromosomes from our biology classes—those paired strands in the

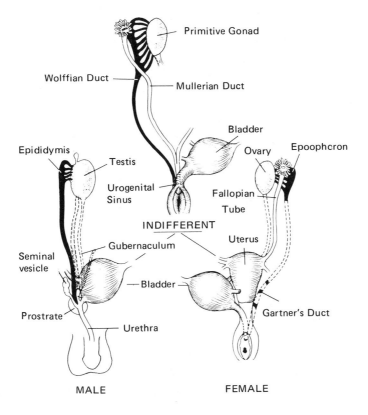

Fig. 3–12. Influence of steroids on differentiation of the male and female sex organs from the primitive rudiments.

nucleus of each cell that determine whether a child will be born blue- or brown-eyes, or club-footed. Mature human *germ* cells, ovum or sperm, contain one -half of a complete set of chromosomes: 22 autosomes and one sex chromosome. The sex chromosome in the ovum is always a single X chromosome, one of the *somatic* pair XX. However, of the sperm cells, half contain a single X chromosome, while the other half contain a single Y chromosome, one of the *somatic* pair XY. During fertilization, each chromosome of the ovum combines with one chromosome of the sperm to form new pairs: 23 pairs in the case of a fertilized human cell. Now, in this process of fertilization, it is purely a matter of chance whether a female germ cell, carrying a single X chromosome, will combine with an X-bearing or a Y-bearing sperm cell, i.e., whether the child will be a girl or boy. (Fig. 3–13.)

This was not always the case! The simplest organism, such as a bacterium, reproduces by duplicating its complete set of chromosomes before dividing into two *identical* daughter organisms. Because of this duplication of the genetic material, the "mother" organism's characteristics are preserved in all of its descendants. These so-called clones have the disadvantage that they cannot readily adapt to changes in their environment. This condition improved as organisms continued to climb the evolutionary scale. Then two *different* individuals each supplied one half of analogous sets of chromosomes, which united to form new genetic variations. Even so, the offspring still lacked the specifically male or female orientation whose advantages we pointed out.

How did this sexual differentiation come about? There are several theories, offering possible explanations. At any rate, it seems that—some 200 or 300 million years ago (or was it 500?)—a new, small chromosome appeared. This Y chromosome in some cases, replaced one of the older X chromosomes. In the manner described above, fertilization resulted in organisms whose sex chromosome pair (in humans, the twenty-third pair) did not always consist of identical mates. Those whose genetic material included the combination XY are called male. Their Y chromosome (or perhaps the absence of the second X chromosome) causes an acceleration of androgen production. The XY combination probably does not induce hormone production directly but, rather, stimulates development of the appropriate secretory cells. As early as four weeks after fertilization (prior to appearance of the female sex hormones), the XY organism is already synthesizing its first sex hormone, which happens to be testosterone—a male hormone. Thus, the male has won his first victory, which some people claim that is his last!

By this *coup de main,* testosterone causes regression of the Müllerian ducts (which would soon have started to develop female organs and hormones), of which nothing but remnants are left in the male. Instead, the Wolffian ducts and the cloaca are stimulated to grow. Unrestricted by estrogen, a typically male sexual apparatus is formed in contrast to the indistinctive structures of the bisexual organism. Also, without estrogen inhibition of testosterone production, the absolute hormone level in the blood becomes higher than in bisexual animals.

Moreover, the target organs are sensitized so that later on, during puberty, they will preferentially respond to the same androgenic hormones that have created them. In addition to the primary and secondary sex organs, the muscles and skeleton and, in particular, the brain are sensitized as well. Already at birth, the brain of the XY organism is formed irrevocably male to such a degree that differences in behavior between boys and girls at play can be attributed to environmental influences to a limited extent only. According to the most recent research findings, testosterone in the embryo determines the "wiring" among individual brain cells in such a way that subsequently administered female hormones, even in massive doses, can no longer have a feminizing psychological effect.

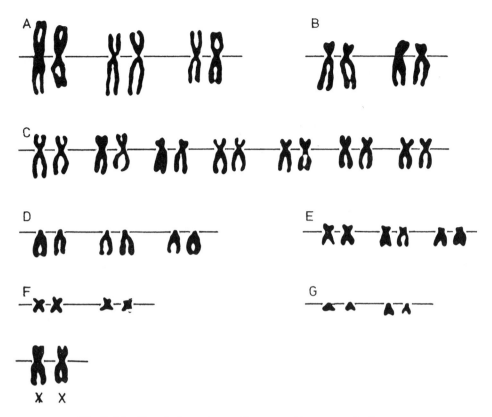

Fig. 3-13. Female karyotype, diagrammatic representation.

The opposite happens when two X chromosomes are combined in the fertilized cell. During the eighth week of gestation, while testosterone production is delayed, massive amounts of estrogens are produced, causing deterioration of the Wolffian ducts so that only remnants are retained in the female reproductive system. Instead, the estrogens, uninhibited by testosterone, stimulate the Müllerian ducts to form the female sexual structures so that a female embryo develops. Here too, in comparison to bisexual animals, we find increased hormone production and development of target organs, such as the mammary glands and the uterine endometrium, which will later respond to increased amounts of female sex hormones during puberty.

In summary, polarization during the *first* phase results in increased plasma levels of the respective hormone, inhibition of the contrary hormone, development of gender-specific organs, and hormone sensitization of these and other structures.

Of course, the actual process of sexual differentiation is much more

complicated than that. However, the principle prevails: a minor time difference in the onset of production of one or the other steroid is the snowball
which starts the avalanche of divergence in either direction. It sounds
incredibly simple and is, moreover, accomplished extremely efficiently. Only
seldom does something go wrong in this process, producing an individual
whom we call a hermaphrodite.

After the steroid hormones had accomplished the task of separation, they
started to tackle the second problem by preparing for the *union* of the
sexes—this time without any help from the chromosomes. The sexual apparatus required for fertilization, sensitized to begin with, is brought to full
maturity during puberty through the influence of either testosterone or
estrogen. We might call this the sexual action of the steroid hormones.

From an evolutionary point of view, mating behavior presents some difficulties in that two individuals of intentionally different natures must find
each other attractive in order to make fertilization possible. Once again, the
sex hormones solve the problem elegantly. During puberty, when their
sexual action causes changes in hair distribution and voice quality, as well as
the development of feminine "curves," these hormones simultaneously sensi-
tize the preprogrammed brains in such a manner that, suddenly, what the
contrary hormone created is perceived as beautiful. Overnight, the "trouble-
maker" and the "silly goose" turn into Romeo and Juliet, without any
changes that might be noticed by the objective observer. Here, we are experi-
encing not a sexual, but rather a cerebral action of the hormones.

The wisdom of the old Arab saying that "beauty lies in the eye of the
beholder" becomes evident. This applies not only to man but to the entire
animal kingdom, governed by the same laws everywhere, and is a source of
beauty and admiration. We may ask ourselves why there is such agreement
among vertebrates on what is perceived as beautiful. It is strange and makes
us wonder, since it does not follow naturally that we should perceive as
beautiful the changes brought about in animals by androgens and estrogens.
After all, why should a human being take pleasure in the magnificent display
of the peacock's tail, the nuptial plumage of the orange weaver finch, or the
grace of the doe? Yet, they are also experienced as beautiful by humans.
Then again, this may not be so surprising if we bear in mind that all these
changes are caused by the same steroid hormones for which the human
being too is sensitized.

It is true, however, that not all ideals of beauty are generally appealing.
There is yet another, very peculiar mode of hormone courtship which, rather
than stimulating the mate through the intermediary action of physical
beauty, directly triggers nervous responses, often over large distances. Such
remote-action hormones are called pheromones. The better-known phero-

mones are those that attract butterflies over great distances. Among the steroids, there are only a few pheromones and, therefore, we will mention them here. A hundred years ago, Louis Agassiz observed that female crabs, helpless for a few days while molting, are embraced and protected against enemies by male crabs. Ryan found, in 1949, that the male crabs are attracted, and their behavior incited, not by the visual appearance of the females, but by a steroid hormone (pheromone) secreted in the female urine at molting time which acts directly on the brain of the male. Another example of an experience of beauty that we cannot share is the scent of $\triangle^{16}$-androstene which hogs secrete through the salivary glands, and whose musky odor elicits sexually receptive behavior in sows.

After all we have learned, very little remains to be added with regard to the *third* phase, synthesis. Man's protective, and woman's nurturant behavior are ensured by characteristics which simultaneously serve to enhance mutual attraction. Man's body size, his aggressiveness and his strength are consequences of testosterone action on the brain and muscles. On the other hand, a woman's caring nature, the development of mammary glands and a fat cushion for "times of need" are due to the effects of female sex hormones.

We must pause here, for a moment, to fully appreciate the masterwork nature created in sexualization, not only in terms of implementation, but also from a conceptual point of view. Out of one individual, nature has created two physically separate beings who need each other in order to guarantee their perpetuation. She has accomplished this miracle with a minimum of expenditure, through the skillful manipulation of certain components whose remnants, without exception, are still in existence: every man still possesses traces of female hormones and, conversely, there is testosterone in woman's blood. Both sexes respond to follicle-stimulating hormone (FSH) and luteinizing hormone (LH), and both still retain vestiges of the Müllerian or Wolffian ducts, respectively.

Summing up this hypothetical development, we have established that the chromosomes, while providing the initial stimulus for sexualization, contribute nothing to its specific manifestation. Consequently, they do not determine the difference between the sexes. The same is true for the gonadotropins. They are present to the same extent in both sexes, even though subject to different rhythms of production. By no means, however, do they influence the difference in appearance between man and woman. This means that *la différence* is due solely to the action of the steroid hormones.

A long journey, starting out with the experiences of Greek peasants and continuing through Berthold's experiments, was necessary before this conclusion could be reached. At first, it was empirical observation that pointed toward the existence of sex hormones, then came their postulation and finally, in 1929, proof of their existence was established. That was almost 50 years ago. Adolf Butenandt, who, in 1929, discovered the follicular hormone, is still active because he was so incredibly young when he achieved success. Very few people enjoy the good fortune of being able to experience what has become of the fruit of their labor. One would like to meet one such person.

I am early for my appointment and stop the car at the little cemetery, Martinsried, on my way to the Max-Planck Institute. The warmth of the intense April sun is modified by a crisp breeze. Between the silent, somewhat old-fashioned headstones lies the grave of a soldier born in 1929. There have been revolutions since then, and wars, but in the long run, the events of that year will prove to be of greater significance.

Soon, I recognize the bizarre, cube structures of the Institute amid the Upper Bavarian countryside. It takes a little while to find Butenandt. "The professor? Your best bet is the hallway straight ahead"; the doorman scratches his head and then changes his mind: "No, you'd better try building D, one flight up." In the end, it turns out to be the ground floor after all.

The impression of a friendly patriarch hovers over the long hallways, lined with small labs and offices. In the last office, I find a tall, lean, white-haired man, with a scar on his chin. Assuming, for a moment, that I were un-aware of being face to face with one of the great men of this earth—the discoverer of follicular hormone, androsterone, progesterone, ecdysone, a Nobel Laureate, a knight of the order Pour Le Mérite, honorary president of all Max-Planck Institutes—I would still be able to sense it. This must be Adolf Butenandt.

He sits in the morning sun, enjoying his cigarette, and tells about the circumstances surrounding the discovery of the follicular hormone. He speaks, full of enthusiasm and without melancholy, of those years which are the most memorable of our lives because we were so filled with illusions. The atmosphere of the Chemical Institute at Göttingen comes to life again. Monastic dedication to work was modified by excursions into the Harz Mountains and frequently ended over a glass of wine with the chief. Butenandt tells of the fateful day when Windaus charged him with the investigation of the sex hormones without realizing, at the time, that they were steroids. The order originated from a pharmaceutical company, and it was by lucky coincidence that it went to Göttingen. Windaus, who was busy with the cholesterol problem, assigned the project to his young assistant.

Again and again, Butenandt searches for the proper words to do justice to his teacher, to express his gratitude and admiration for Windaus' generos-ity and, on the other hand, to acknowledge the achievements of his own assistants in the discovery of the follicular hormone. They mark the true greatness of this man—his humanity, his decency.

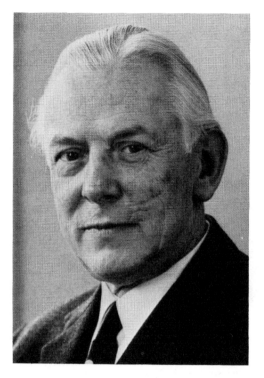

Fig. 3-14. Adolf F. J. Butenandt.

We talk about the events that led up to the discovery of the sex hormones: about Berthold's testes transplant experiments in 1849; about Knauer and Halban who, around the turn of the century, transplanted the ovaries of rabbits and guinea pigs with effects on their vaginas similar to those Berthold had found on the cocks' combs; about their conviction that, in addition to the male hormones, there must be corresponding female hormones which ought to be found in the ovaries. Subsequently, traces were also discovered in the human placenta. On the other hand, there appeared to be little evidence of their presence in the blood or urine.

We talk about the following 20 years of futile attempts to produce effective extracts from these organs, for the same reason that had delayed Windaus' vitamin D work: because there was no quick method of ascertaining whether or not the hypothetical hormone was present at all in a certain extract.

Then, during a visit to Washington, biochemist Edward Doisy heard from a friend, anatomist Edgar Allen, that the mouse might hold the key to the problem. Together they worked out a test, known as the Allen-Doisy assay, that has been indispensable to this day. It involves injecting a mouse with the test substance and subsequently examining the response of its vaginal cells.

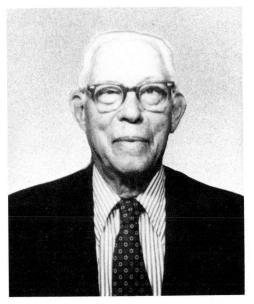

Fig. 3-15. Edward Doisy.

By means of this test, it was possible to determine the presence of as little as .0001 mg of an estrogen.

Although the hormone had not yet been isolated, it was now possible to determine in what extracts it was present and in what concentrations. Slowly and inexorably, investigators began to zero in. The greatest difficulties resulted from the incredibly small quantities that scientists had to work with in attempting to isolate the hormone. At times, they were working with organs that contained no more than ten mouse units per kilogram (kg), i.e., there was one part hormone to one thousand million parts of inert material! How could the hormone possibly be separated?

The decisive turn of events came in Berlin, in 1927, when Aschheim and Zondek found large quantities of the desired hormone in the urine of pregnant women. This was a particularly fortunate circumstance since, not only was urine available cheaply and in unlimited quantities, but also it did not contain any confounding by-products, such as protein or tissue, which had presented so many difficulties in processing ovarian materials. As soon as this fact became known, an international race started on both sides of the Atlantic. Across the ocean, it was mainly Doisy and his assistants who tackled the isolation problem. Europe, however, had a number of experienced people working on it: Laqueur, Aschheim, Löwe, Zondek, and many others. At the time, no one had ever heard of Butenandt, whom Windaus had just assigned to the task.

Doisy, the more experienced investigator, won the race by a head. On

August 23, 1929, during a presentation to the International Physiology Congress, he showed the first two photographs of a crystalline steroid hormone (see Figs. 3–16 and 3–17). The quantity that Doisy recovered weighed 1.39 mg. A few months later, the previously unknown Adolf Butenandt reported that he had also isolated the follicular hormone—after only one and one-half years of work, together with his future wife, Erika von Ziegner. Butenandt, who was only 26 years old, had an idea of the structure

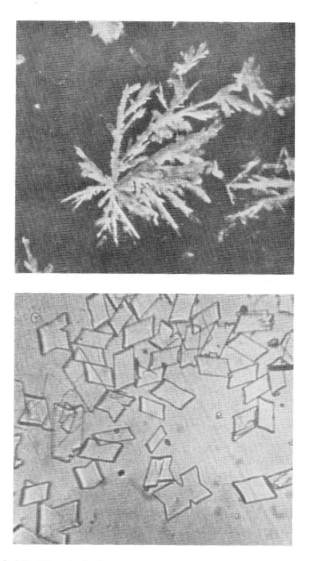

Figs. 3–16 and 3–17. Historical photographs of the first steroid hormone discovered by Doisy (*bottom:* in crystalline form).

even then. In his first publication he pointed out that the new substance was probably a steroid—its relationship to digitalis was obvious to him. However, for the time being, he could not prove it. The structure of this hormone, which was given the name estrone, was later established (see Fig. 3–18).

We talk about Wieland's first, 1928 structural formula of a steroid, which had not been quite correct (see Fig. 3–8) and which had been criticized by Butenandt at the time—for esthetic reasons! "The unsightly corner of the B ring bothered me. I simply could not image that nature was as unesthetic as that." This seems an unusual reason for a scientist whose only measure ought to be expediency. Then it strikes me: to perceive nature's expediency as esthetic is true genius. Anything else is diligence, talent, luck. Any one of us is capable of perceiving the inherent beauty of a crystal or a sunset, but it takes more to appreciate the beauty in the only possible configuration of a steroid molecule.

While Doisy searched for additional estrogens and would, at a later date, reveal the identify of vitamin K (winning the Nobel Prize), Butenandt turned to the male hormone. Again, he was aided by a biological test, Koch's capon comb test: if a castrated cock, whose comb has regressed, is treated with an extract containing the unknown male sex hormone, after two weeks of treatment the surface of the comb and wattles will increase up to six times (see Fig. 3–19).

This time, Butenandt started with urine as a raw material. He received the necessary quantities from police barracks between Berlin and the Balkan peninsula. Tscherning worked with him. Out of 15,000 liters (l), Butenandt finally isolated 15 mg of a male hormone which he named *androsterone*. The year was 1931.

Butenandt analyzed the structure of this hormone and concluded that because of what, at the time, appeared to be an incredible coincidence, he was once again dealing with a steroid (see Fig. 3–20). At a time when all he had on hand was 25 mg of the pure substance, he was ready to propose a formula which could not be proved correct until many years later, when sufficient quantities became available for structural analysis.

However, Butenandt's search had not ended. He then attempted to

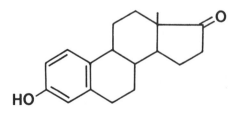

Fig. 3-18. Estrone.

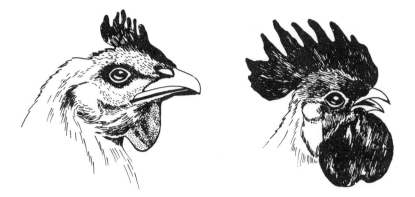

Fig. 3–19. Capon, before and after testosterone treatment.

isolate an additional female hormone which was supposed to differ in its effects from estrogen. The Americans called it progestin. However, to his disappointment, investigation of urine yielded nothing but inactive metabolites, and the amount of active substance found in the blood was insufficient. Consequently, Butenandt began the difficult process of extracting the missing hormone from sows' ovaries. He was not the only one working on the isolation of this substance. The problem had been recognized all over the world, and scientists everywhere were working in high gear to track down the hormone assumed to be in the corpus luteum of the ovaries. The test which, this time, allowed the search to be made had again been developed by two Americans—Comer and Allen. For three years, hormone laboratories in Europe and America worked to tackle the problem, and it appeared improbable that success should once more favor Butenandt.

In our conversation, Butenandt describes vividly how, in the fall of 1933, he arrived at Danzig from Göttingen, a brand-new professor, at age 30 the oldest of a research group of young assistants and students. Only the ovariectomized mice, brought along from Göttingen, were younger. Those must have been unforgettable times for Butenandt and his group: riding on horse-

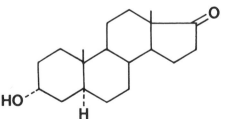

Fig. 3–20. Androsterone.

back through the coastal pinewoods in the early mornings, spending the days in competition with the world's foremost biochemists, and ending at night with a swim in the cold waters of the Baltic Sea. Then, one March day in 1934, he and his assistant Westphal witnessed the formation of glittering crystals in the neck of a retort. "A sight for which we were ready to give a thousand days of our lives!" On April 11, they reported to the German Association for Internal Medicine that they had found the desired *corpus luteum hormone.*

During that year, Slotta in Breslau, Allen and Wintersteiner in the United States, and Hartmann and Wettstein in Switzerland isolated the same hormone. At a conference in London, attended by all concerned parties, it was named *progesterone* (see Fig. 3–21).

The largest quantity of this hormone that Butenandt ever held in his hands, was 20 mg and for that he needed the ovaries of 20,000 sows. He knew that recovery by this method made no sense for therapeutic purposes and found a way to synthesize the hormone from soybean oil. We will appreciate the importance of this synthesis at a later point.

In 1935, last of the important sex hormones, *testosterone,* was discovered. For a long time, androsterone had been considered the actual male gonadal hormone until, in Amsterdam, Laqueur and his research group succeeded in isolating the still more potent testosterone. Within three months, they were able to establish the structural formula, together with Ruzicka in Switzerland and Butenandt at Danzig (Fig. 3–22).

In 1939, Butenandt was awarded the Nobel Prize for his work, but was prevented from accepting it by the German government. Later on, after the War was over, he received the diploma by regular mail, but the money remained in Stockholm.

The first great act of steroid research had ended. Its actors were like comets in the skies of science. Their theme—the bedrock on which our lives rest.

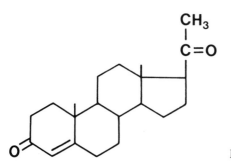

Fig. 3–21. Progesterone.

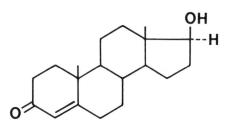

Fig. 3-22. Testosterone.

The consequences of these discoveries were immense. They were not restricted to the field of natural science but have had a profound influence on our outlook on life, much more so than we might realize. It is true that Darwin had proven man's phylogenetic relationship with lower animals, but this did not rule out a special position, a transcendence of self, for man. Now, we were suddenly faced with visible evidence, sparkling crystals, which we not only shared in common with lower animals but which also, supposedly, controlled our behavior and thinking. Suddenly, we were no longer unique, individual beings. This must have engendered a state of shock which was none the less profound for penetrating but slowly into human awareness. After the earth had lost its unique status in Copernicus' times, it was now the human species, our very individuality, that was being challenged. Admittedly, from a philosophical point of view, this step had already been taken some time ago, but there had been no evidence to help it gain acceptance. We should ask ourselves whether the interest in existentialist thought, which has flourished during our times, may have been awakened by these discoveries of the twenties and thirties. Furthermore, to what extent does our present sceptical philosophy of life stem from the feeling of being mere "puppets manipulated by our hormones and nerves." It will take time to get over this second Copernican shock. That will come about as soon as we recognize that these discoveries have simultaneously made us free in a higher sense.

Obviously, we are no less bound by nature's blueprint, no less dependent on the hand of our creator, today than we ever were, but we now have the opportunity to look inside ourselves and to understand ourselves better than we ever could before. In certain cases, we have even been given the chance to correct the flaws in nature's tapestry since, when the sex hormones became available as pure substances, a breakthrough was accomplished, not only in terms of insight but also with a view to potential remedial action. As far as insight is concerned, it came as a surprise to everyone that testosterone, in spite of its name, is also produced in the adrenal cortex and in the female gonads, the ovaries. One is tempted to speculate as to which of the personality traits characterized as typically "female" or "male" may be attributed to this hormonal commonality. Furthermore, it was observed that testosterone accounts not only for the development of obviously male characteristics, such as the dorsal crest of the salamander, but also for behavior unrelated to mating, e.g., the social dominance order of hens that defines those hens that may peck others and those that must suffer pecking. Testosterone treatments result in advancement of an individual hen's position within the pecking hierarchy. This, again, provides a subject for much speculation. Let us consider first the male hormones:

The functions of testosterone (to which we will limit our observations for the time being) may be summed up in three categories: the androgenic or masculinizing effect, which is the most obvious, the anabolic or protein-building effect which is frequently used therapeutically, and the inhibitory effect on the hypophysis.

The *androgenic* effect is rarely used for therapeutic purposes. However, there is a developmental aberration where the testes fail to descend into the scrotal sac from their place of embryological origin, the abdomen. If the situation did not correct itself with time, testosterone treatments used to be prescribed, with surgery the last resort. Why is this condition important? Simply because the abdominal cavity is too warm for the spermatocytes. In order to mature into fertile sperm cells, they need a location that is slightly cooler than normal body temperature.

Then there are children with chromosomal abnormalities whose testosterone production never reaches normal rates and who, consequently, come close to being hermaphrodites. The names of these disorders are unimportant in this context. However, it is significant that androgens frequently represent the only means for therapeutic intervention.

In the normal mature male, administration of androgens is generally restricted to disturbances of libido and potency, which occur with advancing age. Replacement therapy compensates for the body's gradually diminishing testosterone production. A series of testosterone treatments frequently restores mental and physical well-being—unfortunately, however, often without similarly beneficial effects on outward appearance. There is no fountain of youth, but man insists on having his own way, and the question of whether or not to tamper with nature has already been answered in the affirmative by most of us.

In addition, testosterone is prescribed for treatment of certain cases of infertility, where there is reason to suspect a testosterone deficiency. However, in this connection, there is no such thing as dramatic success. As a rule, treatment is drawn out and complicated (for both man and wife) and success still depends a little on the Good Lord's blessings, as people used to put it in the olden days. Later on, this was called "luck," and today it is the "concomitant enzyme pattern." Very likely, they all mean the same thing.

The *anabolic* properties of testosterone are somewhat more frequently put to therapeutic use. In cases of kidney disorders, premature infants, slow-healing fractures, or even for doping of athletes, steroids of this group can be used effectively since they have a favorable influence on metabolism. For women, this entails the disadvantage of masculinization: facial hair growth, changes in voice quality and a receding hairline. Therefore, testosterone is often replaced by other steroids in these cases. There is one disease, however, in which these side-effects are considered negligible, namely cancer. We will learn more about this subject elsewhere.

The third action of testosterone, its *inhibitory* effect on the hypophysis, is hardly ever utilized for remedial application. It is, however, very interesting from a theoretical point of view. As we already learned in the case of vitamin D, the steroid hormones are incorporated into regulatory mechanisms. The inhibitory effect of the sex hormones on the hypophysis is a part of such a regulatory mechanism (Fig. 3–23).

In theory, such a mechanism for testosterone might operate as follows: Let us assume that the hypothalamus sends a signal for onset of puberty

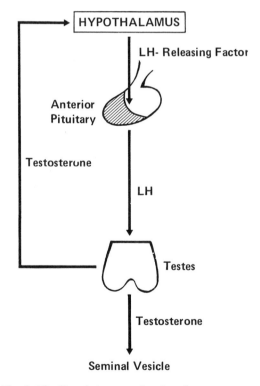

Fig. 3–23. Regulatory mechanism for testosterone.

to the hypophysis, or pituitary gland. The gonadotropic hormone LH is released and stimulates secretion of testosterone. Testosterone, in turn, induces development of the seminal vesicles, stimulates facial hair growth, increases muscle mass, etc. Then the affected organs send a mission-accomplished signal (via the hypothalamus) to the hypophysis. The production of LH ceases and testosterone flow stops.

This is how the feedback mechanism operates for vitamin D, where the *mission-accomplished* signal is integrated into the regulatory cycle. However, in the case of the sex hormones with their multifarious effects, it is impossible to arrive at one single coordinated message signalling the accomplishment of such diverse tasks whose completion is frequently subject to timing differences. Consequently, the hypophysis must make do with a signal indicating an increased testosterone level in the blood. As soon as the intensity and duration of this signal are adequate, the hypophysis, in hopes that all the work has been completed, reduces the release of LH which, in turn, cuts back the secretion of testosterone. It is important, however, to bear in mind that this signal does not indicate successful completion of the actual mission.

Matters are similar in regard to the *female* sex hormones. However, more so than the male hormones, the female hormones have turned out to be fertile territory in our search for self-knowledge as well as therapeutic applications. It was only after isolation of the active substances themselves, that it became possible to differentiate between the various female hormones and their complex actions and interactions. It was found that *estrogens*, including estradiol which is also present in the male body, correspond to the male hormone testosterone in stimulating the development of sex characteristics and maturation of germ cells. After isolation, it became possible, for the first time, to pinpoint the target organs of estrogens (in contrast to progestogens). In addition to the brain, the uterus, vagina and mammary glands all receive specific stimulation controlling their growth (see Fig. 3–24).

Like testosterone, estrogen also has an anabolic function, particularly with regard to bone growth. During puberty (and after a brief lengthwise growth spurt), the epiphysial cartilage becomes completely ossified and no further bone growth takes place.

As we would expect, estrogen has an inhibitory effect on the hypophysis, i.e., on the FSH portion of the gonadotropic hormones. Given this information, we can deduce the corresponding feedback mechanism where, once again, the hypophysis receives a message indicating the circulating steroid level rather than a mission-accomplished signal. (Fig. 3–25)

However, the effects of the second group of female hormones are quite different. The *progestogens*, the most important of which is progesterone, serve to prepare for pregnancy, which has no parallel in the male. Prolifera-

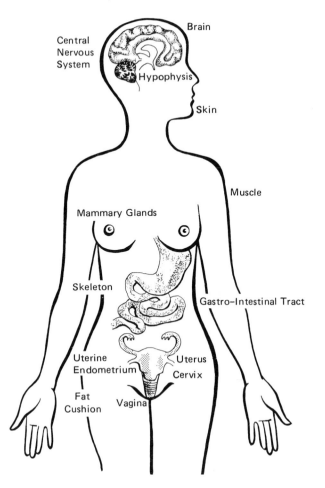

Fig. 3–24. Target organs of the estrogens.

tion of the uterine lining for implantation of the ovum, maintenance of pregnancy and prevention of ovulation are their main effects. Again, there are diverse actions on additional targets such as the liver, the muscles and the brain (see Fig. 3–26). Here, too, we find feedback regulation depending on plasma steroid levels rather than on the effects attained (see Fig. 3–27).

Thus, it finally became possible to understand the female cycle which, up to that time, had always retained an element of mystery. It was discovered how, during the first phase of the cycle, the gonadotropic hormone FSH stimulates growth of an ovum within the ovary, simultaneously activating the production of estrogens. Then, during the second phase of the cycle, the gonadotropic hormone LH brings the ovum to maturation and, at

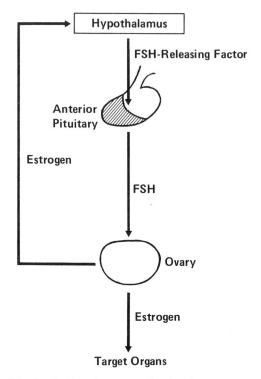

Fig. 3–25. Regulatory mechanism for estrogens.

the same time, initiates progesterone secretion. Figure 3–28 shows a diagram of the female cycle and the release timing of the various hormones during a period of one month.

This is not the place to present a compendium of the various therapeutic applications of the female sex hormones that have become possible due to availability of the pure substances. Out of the multitude of medical uses, the treatment of miscarriage, sterility, dysmenorrhea and menopause—to mention a few—have rescued millions of women from depressing situations (see Fig. 3–29).

The associated methodology has become so sophisticated that medical science has learned, over the past few years, to select medications for each particular kind of therapy in such a way that even the patient's prevailing hormone pattern is taken into account. One particular kind of therapy, however, will be discussed in some detail, since it has probably triggered the greatest biological upheaval since the dinosaur became extinct; that therapy is hormonal contraception.

In order to understand "the pill," we must recall that the circulating

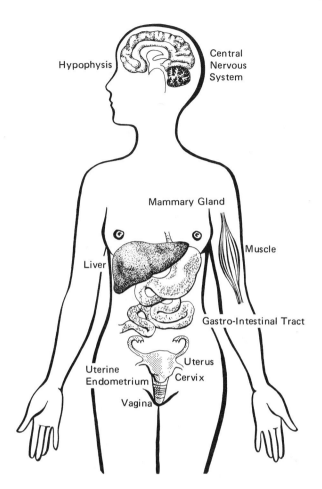

Fig. 3–26. Target organs of progestogens.

steroid level is the only mechanism by which the hypophysis finds out whether or not its instructions have been followed. This represents a sloppy procedure, to say the least. Even for the primary and exclusive mission of the gonadotropins, stimulation of the germ cells, there is no specific measuring apparatus. Whenever the gonadotropins are released in order to bring the ovum to maturation, it takes nothing more than a signal from the circulating steroids to shut down the production of gonadotropins and prevent continued growth of the ovum. It begins to dawn on us what kind of a trick we might play on nature. The first relevant observations came from veterinarians who succeeded in delaying the onset of heat in cows and egg-laying in chickens by implantation of ovaries. Based on these findings, Haberlandt, in Innsbruck,

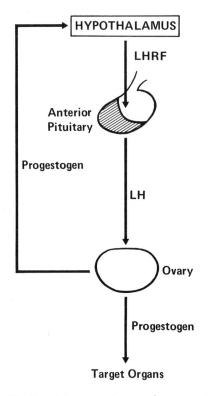

Fig. 3–27. Regulatory mechanism for progestogens.

proposed the equivalent treatment for humans as early as 1921. Incidental clinical observations supported this theory. We will probably never know why a period of 30 years had to elapse before someone turned the idea to use.

The history of these 30 years is very involved—a patchwork quilt of parallel developments whose choronological order is difficult to establish. There was a great deal of overlap, contradiction and repetition. Apparently, the idea of contraception was confronted with a fundamental barrier which seems hardly conceivable to us now and which could be overcome only by a scientist with very special qualities.

The man who possessed these qualities was Gregory Pincus. No one was better suited for this role than the geneticist with the dark, burning eyes and bushy brows, who, together with Hudson and Hogan, and through cooperation from G. D. Searle and Co. and the National Institutes of Health, established the famous Worcester Foundation near Boston. Even while a student at Oxford, he had already been interested in the physiology of reproduction, always with the idea that, somewhere in the long process leading to fertilization of the ovum, he might come across a weak point, susceptible to inter-

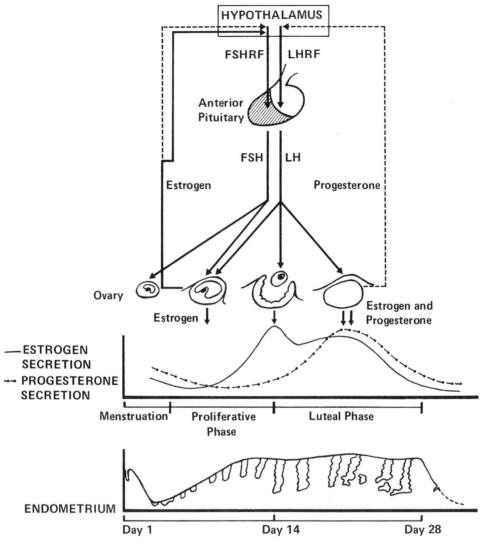

Fig. 3-28. The female cycle.

ference. In the mid-forties, Searle offered him an opportunity to experiment with hyaluronidase inhibitors, substances that were intended to change the consistency of seminal fluid. Since these substances are inactivated when taken orally, Pincus looked for an alternative method and discovered that intravaginal application in fact reduced the number of pregnancies in rabbits. However, this did not satisfy him; he felt that it was more logical to prevent ovulation entirely. Pincus had heard that, according to John Rock of

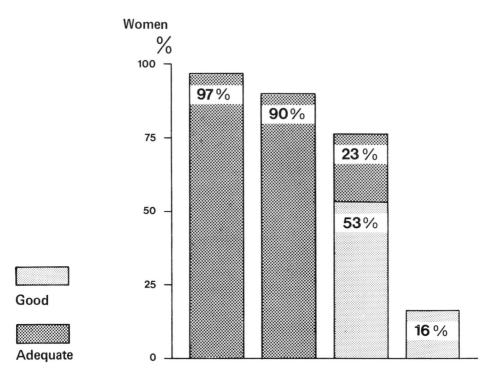

Fig. 3–29. Outcome of treatment of hot flashes in women using estrogen, estrogen + androgen, androgen, and a placebo (double-blind study).

Harvard, who had found the first fertilized human ovum, ovulation was controlled by hypophyseal influence on the ovary. Could this be a point for interfering—for stimulating or inhibiting ovulation? Unfortunately, the involved hypophyseal hormones are proteins as well, i.e., they are destroyed in the stomach and must therefore be administered by injection. This, however, results in sensitization of the patient. Consequently, Pincus had to abandon this route.

Prior to this, Hamblin and Greenblatt had picked up Haberland's idea of ovarian implants, which they refined by using the pure hormone preparations in their animal experiments and, in 1935, Pincus and Chang had succeeded in inhibiting ovulation in rabbits by injection of progesterone. However, at that time, they did not recognize inhibition of ovulation as the final goal; the old problems persistently obscured a clear view.

Assuming correctly that the observed suppression of ovulation had been caused by a feedback effect of the steroids on the hypophysis, Rock and Pincus proceeded to stimulate the hypophysis through a rebound phenomenon—a short-term inhibition by steroids followed, on discontinuation of therapy, by increased activity of the hypophysis. As it turned out, this strategy, known as the "Rock rebound," became an accepted therapy for certain types of female sterility.

It soon became obvious that this principle could just as well be reversed and used to inhibit ovum maturation, which depends on the hypophyseal hormones. All that needed to be done was to apply sufficient amounts of steroids from an external source over an adequate time period, and thus make use of an artificially raised level of circulating hormones to trick the hypophysis into ceasing its activity. As a consequence, ovulation would be stopped as well.

This was recognized by many, but once again the great psychological block interfered with progress. For medical and, above all, ethical reasons, testing with human subjects did not turn into the competitive race that had been expected. Instead, clinical testing started out on a small scale, with Pincus administering daily doses of 300 mg of progesterone to young Puerto Rican women to prevent conception. As month after month elapsed in breathless suspense, his theory was confirmed. However, even though no pregnancies developed, something else did: a high-grade neurasthenia in the patients who, instead of being pregnant, were now suffering from amenorrhea. The absence of menstrual bleeding, unimportant per se, had a catastrophic effect on the participants. In increasing numbers, they abandoned the experiment and, even then, their symptoms did not subside entirely. Then someone remembered (or was it Pincus' idea?) that, as early as 1933, Kaufmann, in Germany, had interrupted progesterone treatment (of an unrelated disorder) for one week every 20 days, which resulted in a monthly bleeding period. It is true that this was not actually menstruation, since there was no ovulation. Rather, it was a so-called withdrawal flow, but it had served its purpose at the time. Pincus adopted the method and, indeed, wives, husbands and investigators were cured of the "amenorrhea psychosis." In retrospect, this idea appears to be nothing more than common sense, but, at the time, it was a milestone for it would make the pill acceptable.

However, for the time being, this method was out of the question for large-scale contraceptive application, since progesterone is destroyed in the gastrointestinal tract and must be injected to ensure its efficacy. Pincus turned to the pharmaceutical industry for advice, and a meeting was called in which Colton from Searle and several chemists from the Syntex company participated. The consensus was that it must be possible to synthesize a progestogen that could be taken orally. Only one matter remained to be settled—which of the many steroids to start out with. After extensive deliberation, the substance chosen was nortestosterone, a steroid that had only recently been synthesized. It was a lucky choice.

To this day, it remains true that one could not have come up with a better starting material. Syntex won the race by a nose (i.e., by three months) with their norethindrone, which was subsequently to be marketed as Norlutin, Primolut N, Noresthisterone, etc. However, the firm did not take advantage of its lead, and Searle caught up with norethynodrel. Together with a number of other steroids, it was turned over to Pincus and Chang who observed that oral administration did indeed inhibit ovulation in rabbits.

Tests with human subjects confirmed this exciting fact. For the first time, a synthetic hormone, taken orally, prevented conception in humans. Pincus continued his experiments with various other steroids and was able to establish that addition of an estrogen in small amounts improved the desired activity and diminished side-effects. However, such a mixed pill could not be put on the market since, according to the rules of the Food and Drug Administration (FDA), combination products were illegal at the time. Moreover, as the date approached on which this product was scheduled to become available, more and more companies disassociated themselves from the project in anticipation of an outraged public's negative reaction to this line of products. In the end, the only firm left was Searle with norethynodrel. For a single-component product, its properties came closest yet to those that others could obtain only by the addition of estrogens. The senior Mr. Searle took personal responsibility for public sale of the drug since he was convinced that he was rendering the world a service.

Meanwhile, the opposition was armed and ready for such a product. The practice shots had been fired. There were even reports that the president of the United States had personally ruled out allocation of public funds for family planning, and public opinion appeared to support him. In 1956, under these adverse conditions, Searle put on the market the world's first oral con-traceptive, norethynodrel, using the trade name Enovid. However, they were careful; the pill was registered with the Food and Drug Administration (FDA) as a "progestational agent" and, in a shrewd move, a conspicuous warning against "possible contraceptive activity" was added.

D-Day arrived, and the few sales representatives, who had not resigned out of depression or on ethical grounds, held on to their hats as they headed for their assigned territories, the new "progestogen" in their sample cases. Surprisingly, except for a few Catholic hospitals cancelling their accounts, nothing happened until 1959 when Searle, now more daring, officially put in a claim for contraceptive activity. The FDA was furious, cited the hazard of cancer (although the drug had previous FDA approval for sale), and refused to accept the claim. A three-hour, heated debate ensued, for which Dr. Winter of Searle had called in Professor Rock, a Catholic, as a specialist for female cancer. Rock reportedly yelled at the FDA's departmental expert:

"What would *you* know about cancer? You talk about religion! What would *you* know about *my* religion?"

This was the atmosphere in which a decision of world-wide significance was made. It is reported here in such detail, because the act of filing the claim for Enovid's contraceptive activity was a signal that indicated man's change in attitude toward the problem of overpopulation. Right or wrong, this move could not be retracted—neither in regard to the method nor in terms of the underlying philosophy. When, in 1960, an FDA committee approved the claim, the battle was over.

Nevertheless, Syntex still hesitated. They granted a license for their norethindrone to Johnson and Johnson who, in turn, set up a new company, Ortho, to market this product as Ortho-Novum. A second license went to Parke-Davis who chose the trade name Norlutin. Gradually, additional companies dared to enter the field, and it was discovered why norethinodrel, a "single-component substance," had obtained such good results: tiny amounts of mestranol contamination had contributed estrogenic effects. Possibly, it was this discovery that led, finally, to FDA approval of combination products.

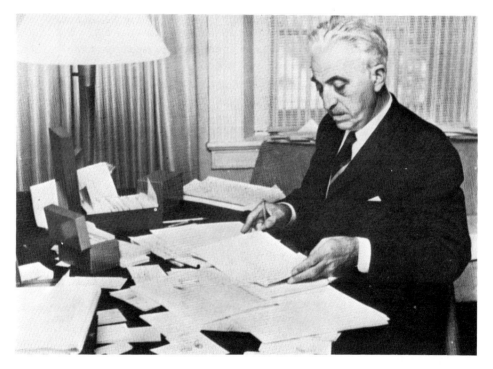

Fig. 3–30. Gregory Pincus.

Over the years, research has come up with three types of pills whose basic principles we should know:

1. There is the combination developed by Pincus, where progestogen is administered for 21 days, always at the same fixed ratio with an estrogen. After discontinuation on day 21, a withdrawal flow follows which the user perceives as menstrual bleeding.
2. Then the so-called phasic preparations were perfected where the progestagen portion is kept low during the first 16 days and is increased to the level of the combination drugs during the following 7 days.
3. Most recently, there has been some experimentation with so-called minipills which contain low doses of progestagen (without estrogens) and must be taken on a continuous basis. These do not inhibit ovulation, and there is true menstrual bleeding. Obviously, in this case, contraception is based on a different kind of mechanism. It is assumed that a hormonal change in the cervical mucus will prevent the penetration of sperm.

All three methods have their advantages and disadvantages and, accordingly, their advocates and opponents. Continued development has not always been directed by purely scientific motives but frequently by the simple desire to administer ever smaller amounts of medication. Since the lowest possible dosages can obviously be achieved only with extremely active steroids, this advantage remains questionable. Nevertheless, considerable progress has been made. In 1951, Pincus was still using 300 mg of progesterone which he subsequently replaced by 10 mg of norethynodrel. In 1961, Searle decreased the dosage to 5 mg and later on, again with the help of a new progestogen, to 1 mg, and even 0.5 mg. For a long period of time, no further dosage reduction could be achieved. This became possible only recently through synthesis of d-norgestrel. Today's minipills contain 0.03 mg. i.e., one-ten thousandth of the original 300 mg.

The search for ever weaker dosages has been gaining momentum due to the much-cited *side-effects* of the pill. Just how dangerous is the pill really? This is obviously an important question since about 20 million women use oral contraceptives. There is no doubt that there are side-effects. However, it is only fair to compare them to the side-effects of pregnancy, to abortions, bleeding, infections and kidney disorders. Viewed in this light, the pill can be less dangerous than pregnancy; nevertheless, it is important to be familiar with its side-effects. It is certainly true that, in a relatively small percentage of women, the pill can cause nausea, headaches, weight gain, breakthrough bleeding and breast engorgement. However, these are relatively trivial complaints compared to the two main accusations—the pill's alleged thrombosis-

and cancer-causing effects. Regarding the latter allegation, it should be stated immediately that it is unsubstantiated as far as the human organism is concerned. This is the conclusion drawn in particular from studies performed by several investigators in Germany. Nevertheless, the experienced gynecologist will recommend periodic examinations for women who are on the pill. Objections regarding the hazard of thromboembolic disease are to be taken more seriously. The unbiased reader of reports published on this subject finds himself confronted with a confusing pile of esoteric statistics and counterpresentations of which even government agencies and pharmaceutical companies can hardly make sense. Yet one might say that an estrogen content of more than 0.05 mg represents a hazard. Most manufacturers have consequently discontinued production of such preparations almost entirely.

These disadvantages must be weighed against the fact that the pill is the safest and most effective method of contraception, apart from the proverbial glass of water. However, it may not be the last word yet. Injections whose effects last for several months, implantation of pellets under the skin, and the so-called annual pill have been undergoing stringent clinical testing for years, as have intrauterine hormone inserts and bracelets that continuously release steroids to the skin.

In all this, it may seem that the male is being neglected. Naturally, it is just as possible to interrupt the hypophyseal-sperm axis by means of steroids as the analogous female mechanism. This has already been done. Experiments using skin implants have shown that it is possible to obtain sterilization for a one-year period by this method.

Now that the underlying principles have been revealed, there is no shortage of suggestions for improvement. In place of pioneers, inventors and innovators, it is now time for diligence and assiduity to take over.

For all the attention accorded this ongoing research activity, we must not forget the prophet of family planning, the man who represented the center point around which this development crystallized. He was not the first to come up the idea of using progestogens for sterilization. Possibly, the trick of interrupting treatment after 20 days, did not originate with him either. Moreover, the pill became a universally accessible drug only because Marker had succeeded in producing progesterone economically from Mexican barbasco. However, it was thanks to Pincus' boldness, to his energetic liveliness which caused him to step on quite a few toes along the way, that the transition from laboratory experiment to the real world was accomplished. The psychological barrier was overcome mainly because of the contributions of Pincus and his Worcester Foundation, and the Family Planning Association of Puerto Rico.

Let us summarize once more, before we conclude this section, the amaz-

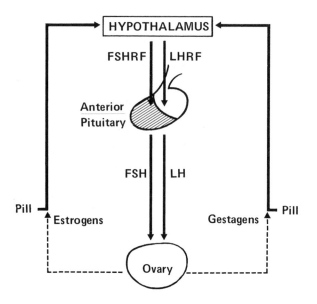

Fig. 3-31. Mechanism of the pill.

ing and cunning idea of hormonal contraception which Pincus developed into a safe and proven method. The gonadotropins, dispatched by the hypophysis to initiate maturation of a new ovum, a new germ cell, are hampered by a blind spot. They have no idea whether or not their efforts have been successful, no idea how much and for how long they must continue to produce to ensure ovulation. As a substitute for this information, they depend on the feedback from another function performed by them, stimulation of the sex hormones. The rising level of these hormones in the blood acts as a signal to the hypophysis, mediated by the hypothalamus, to reduce production (see Fig. 3-31). If this signal is simulated by steroids supplied from an external source, the hypothalamus responds in the same manner and the hypophysis, unwitting target of this underhanded trick, reduces hormone production. Maturation of the ovum in the ovarian follicle is discontinued. Then, since these foreign steroids simultaneously initiate proliferation of the uterine endometrium, the cycle ends with a bleeding phase, as though nothing had happened. The deception is complete.

PROTECTIVE STEROIDS AND DEFENSE

But the living organism uses steroids also for protection. A single low-growing plant occupies a sunny spot at the edge of the woods (Fig. 3-32). From the cluster of velvety leaves rises a tall stem bearing brown-dotted, purple blossoms. For a moment, the serious young man savors the peaceful scene. Then he stoops to dig up the beautiful plant, almost regretfully. He realizes that its leaves are poisonous, but he is unconcerned. After all, his favorite patient only wants the plant as a model for painting.

In the afternoon, when he presents the plant to Helena Cook, she sits up in bed: "Oh, a foxglove! How thoughtful of you, Dr. Withering."

"Digitalis purpurea," he replies stiffly, "of the fourteenth class Didynamia Angiospermia, extremely poisonous, used as an emetic in medieval times. . . ."

Helena does not mind the lecture. She knows that it is for her sake that the young physician takes his long walks. For her sake, he is always searching for different flowers and, now, is even planning to write a book about them. Touched, she picks up one of the leaves of the plant and carefully places it between the blotters of her herbarium: "It will always remind me of you, my dear doctor."

As it turned out, Helena did not need the leaf to remember her physician; within a short period of time, Helena Cook and Dr. William Withering were married. Most of the great medical discoveries had already been made. Withering's compatriots had discovered pulmonary and systemic circulation, had described smallpox, syphilis and the gout, had observed the first leukocytes in the blood. Was there anything at all left to discover?

People tend to search in those areas that they enjoy. Withering, who loved taking long walks through nature's unspoiled regions, believed that, even in the England of George III, there was still something to be learned from folk medicine. Its secret, fascinating potions should be analyzed for active principles, to be applied in accordance with modern medical practice. He therefore decided not to move to the capital city, but to go into medical practice in Stafford. However, no matter how much of his spare time he spent exploring, the results were disheartening: much quackery, much secretiveness, much distrustfulness all around him—but nothing that might be considered world-shaking. Eight years passed before he came upon the first clue to his life's great discovery.

One day, Withering was called to attend a patient suffering from incurable dropsy. A brew, prescribed by an old woman from Shropshire, had caused violent vomiting and diarrhea. Any other physician would have treated the symptoms with laudanum or bismuth salts, or would have been indignant because someone else had been consulted. However, Withering's keen eye took in more than just the toxic symptoms. Amazed, he noted that the diseased body simultaneously excreted large amounts of urine; that the swelling of the legs had subsided; and that the puffing and wheezing, originally his greatest concern, had given way to easy breathing. Absorbed in thought, he ran his fingers through the remains of the tea, saved for his examination by a guilty conscience—roots, a few berries, leaves that he had

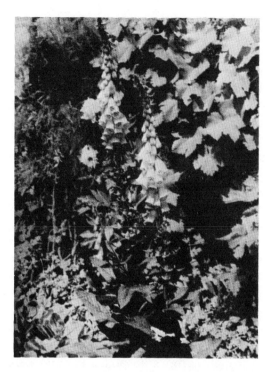

Fig. 3–32. *Digitalis purpurea* (purple foxglove).

seen a hundred times before, Suddenly, he hesitated. He saw himself at the
edge of a woods, digging up a plant, presenting it to Helena. What kind of
plant had it been, and what was there about it that had triggered his memory?

He took the tea home and skimmed through the pages of his wife's
herbarium. There was the entry: *Digitalis purpurea.* In disbelief, he closed
the book. Was it conceivable that this plant, a well-known emetic that had
obviously caused the toxic symptoms, should have additional, unrecognized
effects? Why should it be that no one had previously made this observation?
Withering began researching the digitalis plant thoroughly. To his surprise he
found that Dioscorides, physician of the emperor Nero, had already recom-
mended an herbal remedy, which probably was the foxglove, for treatment of
dropsy. However, in the Middle Ages, this therapy had fallen into disfavor
since the prescription of Dioscorides had brought about vomiting and diarrhea
instead of a cure—although some patients, with God's help, did survive in-
gesting the brew. Careful investigation, claimed the books, had shown that
the foxglove, though not an effective remedy for dropsy, was instead a simple
means for identifying those God protected and those He condemned to perish
as witches. The beautiful plant had become synonymous with trial by ordeal.

One more attempt was made to salvage the foxglove for medicine. In 1542, Bavarian physician Leonhard Fuchs (Fig. 3–33), who gave the plant its Latin name by translating the German word, pointed out its diuretic activity. For a time, the plant became fashionable again, but soon any possible advantages were overshadowed by vomiting and diarrhea. Its administration proved fatal in so many cases that it was little wonder that digitalis was finally condemned by the Académie Française. Ever since then, no reputable physician had dared prescribe it, and neither did Withering—for the time being.

However, the memory of the cured patient kept haunting him. The London *Pharmacopoeia,* England's official book of standard drugs, had irrevocably deleted digitalis from the list of acceptable medications. Could he justify withholding treatment from terminal dropsy patients just because it was forbidden by medical etiquette? Suppose it would be possible to separate the positive effects from the negative ones? Could it be a question of dosage? Was it possible that the diuretic effect, described by Dioscorides and Leonhard Fuchs, might be obtained with a dosage low enough to pre-

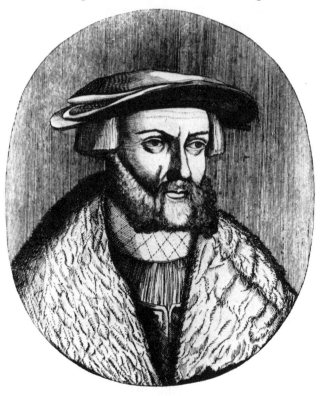

Fig. 3–33. Leonhard Fuchs, 1501–1566.

clude the risk of dangerous side-effects? Or were the two inevitably tied together?

A typical natural scientist, Withering began to experiment. By means of carefully designed tests, he succeeded in proving that what he had assumed was true: the detrimental vomiting was a toxic symptom resulting from high dosage, independent of diuretic action. The only difficulty consisted in preparation of effective extracts without overstepping the narrow boundary between therapeutic and toxic doses. The potency of digitalis preparations varied considerably, depending on the age of the leaves and the season of harvesting. Should the roots be used as well? Should water or alcohol be the solvent? Withering succeeded in overcoming these difficulties and making digitalis safe as a therapeutic agent. This was a great contribution to medical science. Nevertheless, he did not venture beyond his small practice in Stafford just yet.

The great test came when he moved to Birmingham. On July 25, 1776, the physician Erasmus Darwin, grandfather of Charles, officially called Withering in on a consultation. He saw the patient, a hopeless case of dropsy. Without hesitation, he prescribed the notorious medication and, within 24 hours, the patient had eliminated 8 l of water! The medical profession applauded and the case history was published. The breakthough had been achieved. Withering's fame spread all over England and the Continent, even reached distant America. Everyone wanted to meet the famous man, and Withering spent a good number of his remaining years accepting invitations from all over the world, lecturing, consulting and teaching his colleagues the proper application of the new medication. Little did it matter that he did not live to learn that digitalis has no direct diuretic effect (and therefore was not effective in cases of liver or kidney disease). Rather, it acts as a powerful stimulant to the damaged heart and restores its normal functioning. Excessive water retention, or edema, is a symptom of various underlying disorders, one of the most serious being congestive heart failure, where the heart simply does not have the strength to pump out all of the body's fluid intake.

Today, we are better equipped to differentiate digitalis' individual effects on the heart, but this must not detract from Withering's discovery that these effects can be separated through changes in dosage. The smallest dose increases the contractive power of the heart muscle, simultaneously slowing the pulse rate. This is the effect desired in therapy. In this phase, the patient can eliminate between 30 and 40 l of fluid. If the optimum therapeutic dosage (which is different for each individual) is exceeded, the first consequence is an inhibition of the electrical impulse that travels across the heart each second in order to spark its beat. This sparking sequence can be measured

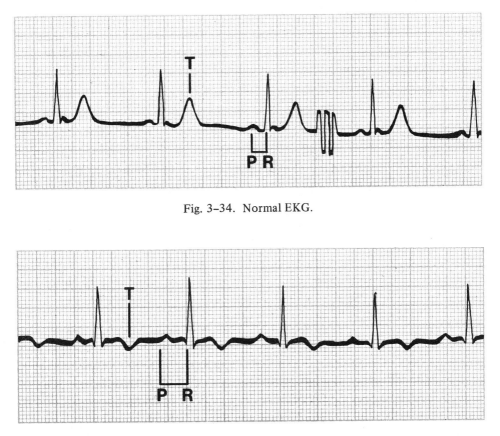

Fig. 3–34. Normal EKG.

Fig. 3–35. EKG after 0.1 mg of digitoxin.

very precisely in an electrocardiogram (EKG). The P-R interval marked in Figs. 3–34 and 3–35 increases from 0.18 to 0.28 second after administration of 0.1 mg of digitoxin. An increased dose of digitalis leads to irregular heart beat, as shown in the EKG presented in Fig. 3–36. Even higher doses cause vomiting and, finally death, which is why digitalis had been discredited in the Middle Ages. Its poison had protected the plant.

These details were unknown in Withering's time, but that was of little consequence. As a single spark can set an entire house afire, his discovery suddenly brought back all the old stories about "poisons" that supposedly promoted fluid elimination. People remembered the squill of the ancient Egyptians, the gillyflower, the lily of the valley, the oleander, the Christmas rose and the old-time hellebore. Even the fantastic superstitious belief of the ancient Chinese, ascribing a miraculous effect to toad skins, was suddenly taken seriously again. There is hardly a country in which they do not grow,

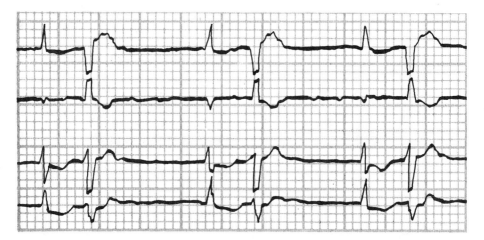

Fig. 3–36. EKG irregularities after increased digitalis dosage.

these plants with poetic names, hardly a population that does not know about their curative (or harmful) properties. There was only one continent where they seemed to be scarce: for a long time, the African arrow poisons were known only for their deadly effect (Fig. 3–37). They were in use all over Africa, spread on the tips of Pygmy arrows and Masai spears. They were employed for trials by ordeal as well as for other purposes. A piece of good advice among bushmen hinted: "A little crushed strophantus rubbed under your fingernails before scratching your friend's back, may save you years of waiting for the pretty widow."

However, the most important use of these arrow poisons was for the hunt. A poison-tipped arrow kills an elephant bull in a matter of minutes. After the wound is cut out, it is safe to eat the meat, since the small amount of poison found in the muscle is scarcely resorbed through the stomach.

Of course, reports of this nature aroused curiosity. Consequently, in 1859, Livingstone undertook an expedition into the darkest regions of Africa. In his party was a botanist, John Kirk, who was to collect samples of these arrow poisons. Kirk was rather careless in handling the poisonous substances, carrying them in the same pocket into which he occasionally tucked his toothbrush. One morning, a little of the poison must have stuck to the bristles and, after brushing his teeth, Kirk suddenly noticed that his pulse was slowing down. He immediately suspected the connection and called out to Livingstone to observe him. Fortunately, nothing further happened. An intact mucous membrane permitted very little resorption and saved Kirk's life. Both explorers concluded correctly that the deadly arrow poison could be used therapeutically, in small doses, to lower the pulse rate. Subsequently,

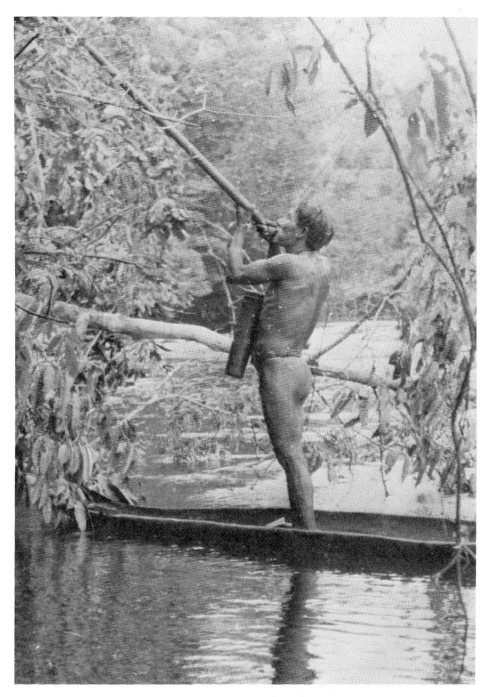

Fig. 3-37. Since time immemorial, steroids have been used as poisons.

Kirk took a jar of this poison, called *kombé*, to England where it was confirmed that this was a cardiac poison, similar in its effects to the foxglove and the squill. Initially, native medicine men refused to divulge the secret of the poison's origin, but it was soon discovered that it was prepared from the seeds of the strophanthus vine. Now Africa, too, had its "poison that promoted fluid elimination."

Once an interest had been awakened, this and the other cardiac poisons were analyzed. With practically unlimited supplies of raw materials, isolation of the active principles was accomplished within a relatively short time. In 1869, Nativelle isolated digitalin from the leaves of the foxglove, with digitoxin and digoxin discovered somewhat later. Fraser was able, in 1870, to extract from strophanthus the active substance ouabain, named strophanthin in Germany. Similar substances were isolated from the remaining cardiac-active plants.

From the beginning, it was recognized that these "poisons" had one thing in common: in the plant, they were linked to a sugar (glucose). They were therefore named "glucosides" or "glycosides." Only the specific component to which the sugar was attached, and which was named "genin," was unknown.

Windaus, in 1915, was the first to suspect that some of these genins might be steroids. As steroid chemistry made progress, the analysis proceeded quickly. To mention all the researchers, who contributed to the work done with the 300 cardiac glycosides discovered so far, is impossible. As their representatives, we should single out Jacobs, Reichstein and, above all, Stoll. Thanks to them, we know the exact structures of these cardiac glycosides and, consequently, their second point in common: *all* of them turned out to be steroids.

Analysis of the chemical constitution of the various steroid glycosides was chiefly pursued by Reichstein and Kuno Meyer. During the course of this work, yet another common feature was discovered. In all of these substances, from one to three sugar molecules are invariably attached at C-3, and cardiac activity is dependent on the presence, at C-17, of an additional five- or six-membered ring with an oxygen atom, projecting at an angle toward the observer. (Fig. 3–38.)

Not all the vegetable *poisons* necessarily affect the heart or the vomiting center in the brain. The potato, for instance, contains the steroid solanine. Is solanine poisonous? Well, this is a touchy question. Some time ago, it was noticed that the Irish, whose diet includes a good deal of potatoes, have a higher percentage of fetuses developing with abnormalities of the spine, or even without heads, than other nationalities. Obviously, this proves about as valid a correlation as there is in Germany between the declining birth rate

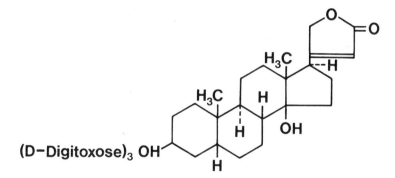

Fig. 3-38. Digitoxin.

and the diminishing number of storks returning each spring. However, the statistical data turned out to be similar for the potato-growing areas in the United States. As a precautionary measure, potatoes containing 1% solanine were declared unfit for human consumption. In 1972, the Social Services Ministry in England even advised women to omit potatoes from their diet during the first few weeks of pregnancy. Meanwhile, matters have calmed down a bit, but the possibility of a teratogenic effect continues to be investigated.

In contrast to the squill, the foxglove, and the strophanthus vine which defend themselves with *cardiac* poisons, solanine represents an example of a steroid's defensive activity that is not directed against the heart of the attacker, but against his *offspring*. In addition, there are vegetable steroids that are *cell poisons* or effective *antibiotics,* such as the tomatine of the tomato. Since scientific research efforts are concentrated mainly on man, the surface has barely been scratched when it comes to investigating the effects of these poisons on plants or lower animals.

Any hobby gardner will have noticed, at some time or other, that the buds of certain plants will continue developing, regardless of heavy mite or aphid infestation, while the delicate neighboring petals have long since withered. The buds of these plants are so chock-full of steroids that it is difficult to isolate them all, let alone identify them. However, it is very probable that the protection these buds enjoy is due to defensive hormones. Some of these act by affecting insect metamorphosis. Also, what applies to the buds is equally true for the all-important seeds. We must ask ourselves what is the purpose of these poisons within the framework of life-sustaining functions that the steroids generally perform? Obviously, the purple foxglove does not produce digitalis to help us.

Although not everyone agrees, there is little doubt that, viewed in the light of their original function, these steroids are *protective hormones* that kill or scare off the robber that eats of them. They represent a powerful means of protection for the many thousands of living things all over the world, which synthesize these substances in their leaves or seeds, in their glands, or elsewhere. Just how powerful this protection is, will become obvious when we consider how the African medicine men locate the deadly plants they need for their poisonous decoctions: they search for trees under which lie dead birds and other animals that carelessly sampled the forbidden fruit.

However, why should it be the *seeds* that are poisonous? What protection do seeds need against the birds that are actually supposed to help disperse them? Probably, the birds are nothing but innocent victims of a much more intensive fight for survival. We probably cannot conceive of all the lethal attacks aimed at a tiny seed that is trying to grow. Millions of bacteria pounce upon the welcome prey, the roots of neighboring trees try to penetrate it and suck its life energy, and animals grind it up between their teeth to reach the concentrated nutrients stored within. The seed's countermove appears to involve a group of steroids known as saponins. In a publication dated 1967, Reichstein lists as many as 100 different steroid glycosides of vegetable origin, whose properties are not entirely known as yet. However, those whose working mechanisms are known are deadly and attack the roots of all life processes. In 1 kg of "early" potatoes, there are 180 mg of solanine, which acts as a cholinesterase inhibitor, one of a class of active substances used in the most potent poison gases.

There are differences of opinion as to whether or not this protection is "intentional." Actually, this question is beside the point, since there is nothing in nature that is intentional in the sense in which we understand the word. Nature's intention finds expression in selection. An organism that fails to exploit advantages created by chance will be at a disadvantage compared to its competitors, In this sense, the control of reproduction by the sex hormones is not "intentional" either, nor is the regulation of electrolyte metabolism by aldosterone, a subject covered in a subsequent chapter. Yet, failure to utilize these mechanisms leads to extinction.

If our theory is correct, i.e., if steroids do form a pattern that is woven into *all* life forms, then we should expect to find protective steroids not only in plants but also, in some form, in other living things. Indeed, we need only look around: a water beetle, by the name of agabus, has discovered the toxic effect of cortexolone on fish. When in danger, it can anesthetize the unwelcome attacker by means of a generous dose of this hormone.

In addition, there are the cardiac poisons of the toads. Wieland and his assistants captured 20,000 toads and expressed the secretions of their parotid glands into wads of cotton until they had a sufficient amount to isolate bufotoxin, as it was called. The protection this affords the toad is obvious to anyone who ever saw a cat unwittingly bite a toad and, consequently, throw up. This effect, which recalls digitalis, explains the application of toad skins in heart therapy in ancient China.

Additional examples are offered by the spiny-skinned invertebrates, also called Echinodermata, that live in the ocean. Starfish are the most familiar ones. Echinoderms represent a phylum of the animal kingdom, i.e., they maintain their individuality equivalent to the vertebrates, the arthropods, and other phyla. Phylogenetically, they are ancient and very far removed from us, much further than, for instance, fish, birds, or even crocodiles, all of which are vertebrates.

Yet, in spite of the tremendous phylogenetic distance between them, the little boy at the beach, curiously observing the small animal with five radial arms, and this starfish share something in common: they both have steroids in their cells. However, while they act on the boy to the effect that he curiously picks up the red, five-armed star, they help the starfish to defend itself. Habermehl investigated these venoms and identified five poisonous steroids in the starfish alone. He noted that they resemble the vegetable saponins. They are glycosides, like the plant poisons, and consist of specific steroids linked to a sugar component which facilitates resorption.

The starfish poisons are stored in the glands of the skin; some may cause a skin inflammation in the careless human handling a starfish. If the venom enters the body through a scratch or cut, nausea, numbness and paralysis may be the consequence.

To the starfish, however, the main purpose of its venoms is not defense, but attack. Bivalves, though closing in a flash, are defenseless against a hungry starfish. Its poison paralyzes their adductor muscles so that their valves open to serve the starfish his clam or oyster dinner. These poisons, discovered but a few years ago, have already proved to be potent antibiotics, effective against microorganisms even when greatly diluted.

Examination of other classes of echinoderms turned up additional, powerful steroid poisons. They are used in defense by sea cucumbers, harmless mud eaters that mind their own business and provide the raw material for trepang, a famous delicacy of the South Pacific. When alarmed, the sea cucumber discharges from the skin, or from a gland in the cloaca, a poison that will kill attacking pearl fish in a dilution of 1:1 million. There are even reports that people have been blinded as a result of corneal damage.

Again, we are dealing with saponins, i.e., foam-producing glycosides that destroy red blood corpuscles and can anesthetize a small mammal. The most amazing fact is that, bridging all phylogenetic distances, this steroid is once again very similar to digitalin: an additional five-membered ring with two oxygen atoms is attached at C-17.

These steroids have between 27 and 30 carbon atoms and not only kill microorganisms but also inhibit the growth of cancer cells in certain strains of mice. The idea of utilizing the toxic protective hormones for our own egoistical purposes has prompted an extensive search which may lead to curious discoveries.

The presence of the steroids' protective function in plants, toads, beetles and echinoderms suggest that it represents a very ancient mechanism which we would consequently expect to find in one-celled organisms as well. Sure enough, it was found in bacteria; these are protected against hostile fungi by a steroid called viridin, discovered in 1945 by Brian, and now used as an antibiotic. At first glance, its chemical structure appears comewhat unusual due to an additional ring formation between C-4 and C-6 , but a closer look reveals its steroidal character. Conversely, fungi are protected against bacteria by a number of steroids which have become therapeutically important over the past few years.

In 1942, Wilkins and Harris discovered a very powerful antibiotic, fumigacin, also called helvolic acid, in a variety of the fungus aspergillus. This steroid has proved particularly effective against the dangerous staphylococcus that can cause suppuration, angina, osteomyelitis and sepsis. In 1945, the Italian investigator Brotzu recovered from sewage-contaminated ocean water another fungus, cephalosporium, which secretes an antibiotic later named cephalosporin P_1 and that was also found to be very effective in controlling staphylococci. In Japan, in 1953, Tubaki discovered that monkey dung contained a strain of the fusidium fungus from which he extracted yet another antibiotic, fusidic acid, which, when tested, likewise proved to be a useful weapon against the staphylococcus.

These steroidal antibiotics are particularly important because they may encounter development of resistance to a lesser extent than other kinds of

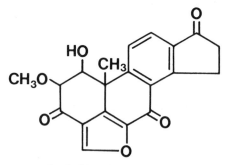

Fig. 3–39. Viridin.

antibiotics. In 1962, the first reports were published about successful treatment of staphylococcus infections in humans, especially osteomyelitis, endocarditis and certain skin disorders that had become resistant to other antibiotics, by administration of fusidic acid derivatives.

Fusidic acid acts by penetrating into the bacterial cell to stop protein synthesis without being inactivated (e.g., as is penicillin) by counter-enzymes. The bacterium can fight back only by developing genetic mutations which prevent *penetration* into the cell to begin with. However, when the *contents* of these "resistant" bacterial cells are exposed to fusidic acid, inhibition of protein synthesis is reactivated. Based on this observation, it appears quite conceivable that, someday, synthetic steroids will be developed which can break through this barrier and against which there will be *no protection.*

In conclusion, we should not neglect to report about a protective steroid that is curious for several reasons. This time, we are looking at insects. An American butterfly, the monarch, has been most thoroughly studied in this respect. It too has protective hormones. What happens when a jackdaw eats this butterfly is reminiscent of the cat and the toad.

Reichstein investigated these emetic steroids, calotropin, calotoxin and uscharidin, which differ only in their sugar component. It is a curious fact that these poisons also grant protection to other butterflies, such as the viceroy, which do not possess them but have gradually developed a coloration resembling that of the monarch. Once a bird has eaten a poisonous butterfly, it will never touch one that looks similar. This indirect use of the protective hormones is known as Bates' mimicry, after the nineteenth century English naturalist. Another strange phenomenon associated with these steroidal poisons is a second form of mimicry: still other butterflies, endowed with poisons of their own, also tend to look like the monarch. They, too, profit from the previous conditioning of the predator and do not have to sacrifice additional individuals of their own to teach the bird what is toxic. This second form of mimicry, named Müllerian mimicry after a German zoologist of the same century, is probably based on the fact that certain warning patterns are more readily recognized than others by the attacker.

For a long time, the third and greatest curiosity in the case of the monarch involved the question of how butterflies—who, like all insects, have lost the ability to synthesize steroids—obtain these protective hormones. It had been postulated that insects acquire their protective hormones from the plants they eat. However, it took more than 50 years before Reichstein and Brown were finally able to prove that the poisonous steroids of the monarch are in fact provided by a plant of the spurge family on which these butterflies feed. Reichstein, moreover, succeeded in presenting similar evidence with regard to an African grasshopper that discharges the same protective hormones as the monarch.

Thus, the insects anticipated a practice that human beings engage in intentionally—exploitation of the protective hormones of other organisms for their own benefit. That may be the greatest curiosity of all.

CORTISONE AND STRESS

The fate of the adrenal glands has been rather extraordinary. Although they are much more important to survival of the individual than, for instance, the sex organs, it was not until the Renaissance that their existence was discovered. This had something to do with the fact that corpses for anatomical studies came from the cemeteries a day or two after burial. By that time, the delicate adrenals were already partially decomposed, with nothing left but flaccid little pouches of tissue which were, consequently, simply called *Capsulae suprarenales.*

Their existence as individual anatomical structures was revealed in 1563. The famous anatomist Eustachio, referring to them as glands, gave a detailed description of the small organs, weighing about 6 g, located at the upper poles of the kidneys (Fig. 3–40).

Even then, discovery of the adrenals was once more delayed by a strange coincidence, almost as though they were trying to remain in hiding. The copper tablets into which Eustachio had carefully and precisely etched his description of the *glandulae renibus incumbunt* disappeared under mysterious circumstances. Only 138 years later were they recovered in the Vatican library and made accessible to medical students.

It is difficult to assess today to what extent this additional delay prevented observant clinicians from detecting, at an earlier stage, some of the amazing relationships involving the adrenals. All we know is that it was not until 1849 that they caught the attention of a physician, the Scotsman Thomas Addison, who was endowed with the keen faculty of observation common to his fellow countrymen. Addison recognized a connection between the adrenal glands and a rare disease he had encountered in some of his patients. They were mostly women between 30 and 40 years of age, whose initial symptoms included fatigue and a dark-bronze coloration of skin areas exposed to light. Subsequently, the fatigue intensified, diarrhea ensued, and the body became dehydrated. While the blood pressure dropped simultaneously, the disease, in its acute form, finally brought death. Because of the characteristic coloration of the skin, Addison named it the bronzed-skin disease.

The discovery of this rare illness had been a difficult project in itself. To

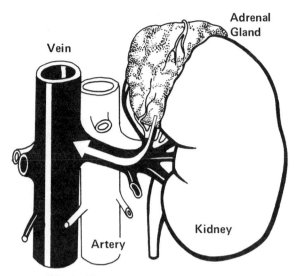

Fig. 3–40. Kidney with adrenal gland.

infer a connection with the adrenal glands was the revolutionary act of a brilliant mind. Until March 15, 1849, when Thomas Addison presented his historic paper to the South London Medical Society, standard procedure had been to start out with the diseased *organ* and look for any associated disorders. For the first time, Addison had started out with the *disease* and looked for the associated organ!

Such a fundamental reversal in the approach to research could not have been accomplished by a man who was nothing more than a keen observer. He also had to have a personality that rebelled against preconceived notions, although, like many other rebels, Addison was distressed by this trait. Even his admirers called him a psychopath. His whole life was over-shadowed by a nerve-racking competition with Bright, successful and sophisticated, and Gull, of noble ancestry, who left an estate of £340,000 when he died and whom no one remembers today. On the other hand, Addison, the scientist, the analytical thinker, a model to his students, remained poor and was always convinced that someone was after his teaching position. Finally, this man of genius ended his life by jumping from a window.

However, no clue to these inner conflicts was reflected in his classic descriptions of diseases. Here the great clinician speaks with self-evident authority. In a monograph which includes pernicious anemia, he describes, based on a mere four cases, the new syndrome that was to bear his name from 1849 on. Who would dare, today, to identify a new syndrome that had gone unrecognized for thousands of years, based on only four case histories and without the benefit of a laboratory? Had there been medical statisticians at the time, they would have had to tear Addison apart, if statistics were to be at all meaningful. However, fortunately, there were none as yet (nor in 1886, when Pierre Marie described his two cases of acromegaly), and "Addison's disease" was born.

It would have been too much to expect that this "comet in starless skies" be immediately acknowledged as such by his contemporaries. He was simply ahead of his time. After the initial flurry of attention, his little booklet of 46 pages just sat there collecting dust in the libraries of scientists who still clung to the organ approach. At the same time, on the Continent, lived a young physiologist, Charles Brown-Séquard, who had read Addison's report attentively. Carried along by the wave of experimentation sweeping across Europe, he attempted to verify the incredible allegations of the English clinician through animal experiments.

While Addison had taken the decisive step forward from description of organs to observation of disease, Brown-Séquard took the next step from clinical observation to controlled laboratory experimentation. He removed the adrenal glands of dogs, cats and pigs, and anxiously awaited the consequent onset of the bronzed-skin disease. Instead, all animals were dead within 12 hours! Suddenly, Brown-Séquard realized that the adrenals play a much more important role than Addison had assumed. The bronzed-skin disease represented only the special case of partial destruction of an extremely essential organ. Its complete elimination spelled death. Without adrenal glands, no mammal could stay alive. There was a singular and astounding revelation—that a wretched little gland, without so much as a discharge duct, should be essential to survival.

On August 25, 1856, when Brown-Séquard read his sensational report at the Académie des Sciences, his colleagues criticized his methods, like anything new that can be subjected to criticism, often justifiably so in regard to details. However, glands that have no efferent ducts of their own became acceptable in the scientific community as of that moment—even though the concept of hormones had not yet entered the scene. Instead, a detoxifying function was postulated. It was assumed that toxic agents were removed from the blood stream as it passed through the adrenal glands. Only through simultaneous advances in sex hormone research did scientists become gradually convinced that, perhaps, the key to the adrenals' vital function might lie not in detoxification, but in *secretion* of an active principle.

The tools of budding chemical science were used to search for these substances, this time with an entirely new objective: therapy. There was a great confidence that this endeavor would be successful within a relatively short time, since miraculous feats had just been accomplished in the isolation of tiny amounts of pigments. If there actually was a substance that could save the victims of Addison's disease, it would soon be available, extracted from the blood (or directly from the adrenal glands). Nevertheless, as much as 40 years later, no such substance had been recovered.

Consequently, there were high hopes when it was finally reported, in 1894, that an English physician had succeeded in raising his own son's blood pressure by means of watery extracts from adrenal glands. Immediately, such an extract was administered to patients with Addison's disease. However, except for an increase in blood pressure, there was no change in their condition. Their fate remained sealed and their suffering could be alleviated only by ingestion of large quantities of common salt. What a profound disappointment!

Scrutiny of the English extract revealed that this involved an entirely different hormone which is produced in the adrenal *medulla*—adrenaline. Only then was it concluded that the desired hormone might, instead, be found in the adrenal *cortex*. An inner gland which produced the newly discovered adrenaline was, so to speak, wrapped in an outer gland containing the hormone that could save the victims of Addison's disease. Yet this hormone of the outer, "wrap-around" gland persistently eluded detection. Over 70 years had elapsed since Brown-Séquard's experiments, and researchers investigating other endocrine glands had been successful with their watery extracts. After adrenaline had been discovered, Banting and Best had found the insulin of the pancreas, and Kendall the thyroxine of the thyroid gland. Even the first sex hormones had been tracked down, but the hormones of the adrenal cortex did not divulge their secret. It seemed obvious that they must be water-soluable, since they were soluble in blood plasma; so they had to be extractable with water. Nevertheless, all watery extracts turned out inactive. It was a complete mystery.

In 1930, based on Rogoff and Stewart's experiments with glycerine extraction, two investigators, Swingle and Pfiffner, speculated that the hormone being sought might be a substance similar to cholesterol, i.e., circulating in the blood, yet not water-soluble. Moreover, they suspected that to obtain any effect might require much larger quantities of the extract than previously assumed. (Today we know that the extractable hormone content of an adrenal gland is so small that it is sufficient for only a 10-minute period of secretory activity. To produce its physiological effects, the adrenal gland must, therefore, produce its own capacity more than 8000 times over a 24-hour period!)

Consequently, two changes were necessary; water could no longer be used for extraction, and much larger quantities of adrenal glands were required. Swingle and Pfiffner, interpreting the implications correctly, applied a method that was revolutionary by current standards: utilizing the adrenals of not two or three, but 350 cats, they extracted with *alcohol* and came up with the first active extracts.

However, these first extracts were far from perfect. One year later, young George Thorn of Buffalo began working out a *standardization* procedure. This was more important and more difficult than would seem at first glance. The problem was that hormone content fluctuated considerably from one batch to another. To an Addison's patient, whose life was in the balance, a concentration that was too low meant death in spite of the injection. On the other hand, an excessive dose of such a crude extract entailed the risk of unpredictable side effects.

Thorn did not talk much, but in 1932, he was scheduled to appear, accompanied by two cats, at the annual convention of the American Medical Association (AMA). He was to present a paper disclosing that he had produced an extract which, when injected twice daily in doses of exactly one unit each, could keep two adrenalectomized cats alive indefinitely. But how could he manage to transport the experimental animals to New Orleans? It was a long trip. Eventually, young Dr. Thorn, his heart pounding, sat in the baggage car of a swaying train, praying, changing trains, and periodically injecting "cortin" into two felines gone hysterical from the long train ride. "When I think of the illustrious audience awaiting me in New Orleans, only to see me arrive with two dead cats, I still have nightmares even now," he related as much as 40 years later. Of course, everything went well. When the young man had completed his presentation, he received a standing ovation and was awarded the gold medal of the AMA. This marked the official confirmation of adrenal therapy as accepted medical practice. For the first time in thousands of years, the bronzed-skin disease was no longer fatal. This represented a great victory on the clinical front.

On the other hand, as far as the chemist is concerned, a crude extract is rather dissatisfying. The chemist wants to know precisely what he is dealing with. He wants to isolate, crystallize, and then, with a sense of satisfaction, solve the puzzle of the formula.

Thus, scientists in the United States and Europe competed to clarify the nature of this extract. On the American side, it was chiefly Edward C. Kendall and his group who actively pursued adrenal research. Kendall's ancestors had immigrated to New England from England and Scotland in 1636, and their descendant, as a young man, had already isolated the hormone of the thyroid gland. However, he was not satisfied to rest on his laurels. In the early thirties, Kendall heard that the adrenal glands were supposed to contain another hormone in addition to adrenaline, a hormone that might save the life of Addison's patients. He had not the faintest notion as to the identity of this substance that prolonged the lives of dogs whose adrenal glands had been surgically removed. Up to this point, only one important fact had been determined: that this hormone was present not in the adrenal medulla, but in the cortex. Therefore, it was tentatively called "cortin." Any chemist with even an ounce of ambition eagerly attacked the task of tracing this "last hormone" that remained to be discovered. Thanks to the tools available to modern chemistry, it should be possible to isolate this substance within a few years.

Great quantities of adrenal glands were required to produce extracts. Kendall, who worked at the laboratory of the Mayo Foundation, found a way to procure these huge quantities free of charge. He told Parke-Davis, distributors of adrenaline, that he would isolate this substance for them from adrenal medullae if he could keep the adrenal cortices in exchange for his work. Parke-Davis agreed. This gave Kendall a decisive lead. Between 1934 and 1949, his group processed 150 tons of adrenal glands. While he was producing adrenaline worth $9 million, he was simultaneously saving $200,000, the purchase price of the raw material needed for his research.

Looking at these piles of hamburger-like chopped adrenals, Kendall racked his brains, at first to no avail, trying to figure out how he could possibly induce them to yield a few crystals of the powerful hormone that could save Addison's patients and adrenalectomized dogs from certain death. By progressively improving the available methods and continuously testing hundreds of extracts in dogs, Kendall and his associates gradually succeeded in isolating five different compounds, all of which had some effect on the adrenalectomized dogs. Using the sequence in which they were discovered, he named them compounds A through E. The exact compositions of these compounds were still unknown, and there was only one method of measuring their potencies which were subject to daily fluctuations: observing their effects on the dogs. The dose required to save the life of one dog was called one "dog unit" but, of course, it varied depending on the dog's diet, its weight and the salt content of its food. The result was an unholy confusion whenever individual laboratories from all over the world tried to communicate with one another regarding the potencies of their respective extracts.

Even after six years of intense effort, Kendall had not come a great deal closer to isolation of the wanted hormone. He could not even say with certainty which of his extracts contained the elusive hormone or whether, perhaps, it was present in each one of them, with the differences attributable to varying concentrations. His disappointment mounted when, in 1936, news leaked out that, beyond the ocean, his friendly rival Reichstein had isolated as many as seven substances, which he had likewise identified by using the letters of the alphabet, only in a different sequence. This was the beginning of a few years of confusion until it was established that, for instance, Kendall's compound E was identical with Reichstein's Fa, and Pfiffner's compound F. For years, the differences in designation were a source of annoying inconsistencies throughout the international scientific literature, to say nothing at all of the bewilderment they engendered in medical students.

Soon, one of Reichstein's extracts, compound H, turned out to be particularly active and, for a while, Kendall was afraid that Reichstein might have succeeded in isolating "cortin." He came close to giving up, since the Swiss chemist's lead appeared unbeatable. Finally, however, after extensive deliberation, he decided to continue his endeavor, influenced by three factors. His singular supply of adrenal glands was probably much greater than the amounts the Dutch firm Organon could ever transport to Switzerland for Reichstein. Moreover, the hormone as such had not yet been unequivocally identified. Finally, and this was his most important reason, Kendall realized that he had already discovered Reichstein's compound H some time ago, albeit identified by a different letter! The only difference was that his extract had simply not been sufficiently concentrated.

Kendall summoned up his spirits and, soon, the balance tipped once more in his favor. He was able to demonstrate that his compound E was convertible into an androgen through certain chemical alterations. This was an immensely important discovery, providing the first clue that cortin probably was a steroid. From this moment on, it became possible to take advantage of all the knowledge previously accumulated about steroids. Without delay, Kendall attempted to approach the search for the mysterious hormone from this direction by utilizing bile acids for synthesis of substances that would produce effects similar to his five original compounds. He established that cortin-like activity was dependent on the presence of an oxygen atom at position C-11 of the steroid. However, once more, Reichstein was able to restore a state of equilibrium. In 1937, he succeeded in producing the first synthetic adrenocortical hormone. He named it desoxycorticosterone acetate (DOCA). Then, inexplicably, Reichstein abandoned steroid research for a while, turning his attention to other subjects, possibly because he believed that he had found "the hormone" of the adrenal cortex.

However, the physiological activity of DOCA was limited to control of the mineral, or electrolyte, deficiencies in patients with Addison's disease, as well as in adrenalectomized dogs, while it had no effect on the disturbances in carbohydrate metabolism. As early as 1932, the physician Britten had warned against focusing exclusively on mineral metabolic activity in the search for this hormone. He believed that carbohydrate metabolism played an important role as well. In line with this warning, it was ascertained through clinical testing, in 1937, that desoxycorticosterone (DOC) could not be identical with cortin. To make matters worse, it turned out that DOCA was not altogether harmless as a medication. As a consequence of the clamor for the new hormone created by sensational news reports, several patients treated with this drug died from salt retention or high blood pressure. Then came the first voices claiming that there was no such thing as "cortin" and that, instead, the adrenal cortex secreted several hormones. Possibly, DOC was the hormone controlling mineral balance, but then there had to be an additional hormone affecting carbohydrate metabolism.

It was 1940 by the time Kendall found out that such a substance probably did exist and that it had to have an oxygen atom at C-11. His compound E seemed to satisfy this requirement. Moreover, he discovered that the un-crystallized residue of his extracts contained a substance whose mineral metabolic activity was greater than that exhibited by DOCA, and which probably contained the true mineralocorticoid hormone. However, he did not pursue this trail, and many years were to elapse before this hormone would, someday, be isolated in England.

Meanwhile, Kendall placed his bet on the carbohydrate-active hormone, assuming that it was present in his compound E. Then came the war and, with it, rumors about U-boats, German submarines which were supposedly transporting adrenal glands from Argentina to Germany—rumors that were entirely without foundation. Nevertheless, the army and navy established an urgent three-point program in which, based on these reports, compound E was given priority over penicillin and the antimalarial drugs. Elsewhere in this book (p. 173 ff.), we will learn how this eventually led to partial synthesis of the steroid hormones. Nevertheless, as far as Kendall was concerned, this research program initially represented a detour. Although it was believed that the Germans were probably developing compound E, there was a consensus that the easiest way to accomplish this was via compound A. The project was assigned to Kendall.

He began, in cooperation with U.S. Merck (Rahway, N.J.), to process several kilograms of desoxycholic acid in order to obtain a substance whose activity would be similar to compound A. However, failure followed upon failure. To make matters worse, his most valuable assistants were drafted. The air of frustration reached a high point in 1943 when Reichstein, who had returned to steroid chemistry, reported that he had synthesized compound A. It would be merely a matter of months before he produced compound E as well. Consequently, the national Research Council terminated the research project. Penicillin had been discovered, and the antimalarial compounds as well, but with the war almost over, American scientists had been unable to produce compound A, let alone compound E. It is not difficult to imagine the level of morale among the participants. Most of the chemists and contributing firms discontinued work on the hormone project; that is, all of them, except for Kendall and the men from Merck.

This obstinate refusal to quit yielded a first glimpse of success in 1945, when the group was able to recover ten times the amount of compound A from the same quantity of adrenal glands as Reichstein used in Switzerland. Yet, clinically, it proved to be a failure. At that point, even the clinicians gave up on the adrenocortical hormones.

Kendall and Merck, however, did not throw in the towel. They established the fact that compound E had to have an oxygen atom at C-17 and a double bond in ring A. Using this structural concept, they continued working, day after day and year after year. Finally, on April 29, 1948, they held in their hands a few grams of this substance which, they believed, had been worth all the efforts of these 18 years.

Unfortunately, by that time, no one wanted any part of compound E. Interest in its potential applications had ceased. Kendall recalls this as the most depressing moment of his life. Months went by, and nothing transpired that might have raised his spirits. Then, one day, a physician requested the entire available supply of compound E for an illness which had nothing to do with Addison's disease. Later on (p. 100 ff.), we will find out how this came about. All we need say at this point is that this telephone call rescued Kendall for a condition which, in a deliberate understatement, he describes as "worry, frustration and anxiety." Wholeheartedly, he seized this last, desperate chance to make something meaningful of the previous 18 years. He invented method upon method for grinding up the new substance, while safeguarding its sterility for injections in arthritic patients. Absorbed in his work, he tried to forget that he had turned 62 and that the Mayo Foundation was planning to phase out his beloved research.

On April 20, 1949, when the Mayo Clinic announced the successful application of the new medication for rheumatoid arthritis, the days of darkness were over. Kendall's star of fame was rising, and he was showered with praise, honors and even more work. This included the assignment of finding a suitable name for compound E, since shrewd operators were already starting to sell vitamin E as a remedy for arthritis. On July 1, 1949, in the ballroom of the Waldorf Astoria Hotel, compound E was officially named cortisone, a name destined to become world-famous. In addition, another decision was made. Kendall, realizing that with all his patents he could become a rich man, thought of all the pathologists, physicians, physiologists and biochemists who had no chance of establishing proprietary rights for their work. Therefore, in a great humane gesture of good fellowship, he waived his rights in favor of the Mayo Foundation. In 1950, Kendall, his great rival, Reichstein, and Hench were awarded the Nobel Prize.

At this point, it is appropriate to pause for a moment to talk about Thadeusz Reichstein, born in 1897 in Poland, son of a Russian merchant, who became the world's greatest expert in corticosteroid chemistry. He is still active at the Chemical Institute of the University of Basel. A casually elegant, live wire of a man, he is not as proud of his accomplishments as of the fact that a rare variety of fern, which he discovered on the isle of Corsica, was named after him.

"When I started investigating the adrenal extracts," he relates, "I was convinced, from the very beginning, of two things: that I was dealing with a *mixture* of hormones and that, this time, they could definitely not be steroids. Regarding the second point, the assumption soon proved false: due to a relatively high oxygen content, this new, previously unknown group of substances was water-soluble to a higher degree than the known steroids. But very soon, we recognized our error." By 1938, Reichstein and his group had isolated 29 different substances from adrenocortical extracts and clarified their structure—all were steroids!

"This work proceeded so quickly because, a few years earlier, the correct structures of various steroid hormones had been established by Windaus, Wieland, Butenandt, Laqueur, and Ruzicka, so that a comparison with substances of known configuration was possible," he acknowledges appreciatively. In 1937, he succeeded in synthesizing the first adrenocortical hormone without realizing it. While attempting to produce one of these hormones, corticosterone, he was unable to attach the necessary oxygen to the C-11 atom of the steroidal skeleton. He therefore named the resultant substance desoxycorticosterone. A short time later, this was discovered among the hormones of the adrenal cortex (all of which, by the way, are called corticoids). However, this hormone, though effective in restoring electrolyte balance in patients with Addison's disease, has no influence on the disturbed carbohydrate metabolism which, initially, was of greater concern to the clinician.

Reichstein continued to discover and synthesize additional steroids, generally by starting out with cholesterol or one of the bile acids. Eventually, he even succeeded in maneuvering the all-important oxygen atom into the famous C-11 position, thus producing Kendall's compound A which he named corticosterone. However, his process was worthless for practical purposes; the few milligrams produced were barely sufficient for a single injection. For a long time, Reichstein had been aware of the fact that the process of synthesis would be child's play if he could only find a suitable, naturally occurring raw material—just one single steroid endowed with an oxygen atom in the C-11 position. One day, he heard of two cardiac-active glycosides which were supposed to satisfy this requirement. One of these was produced from the foxglove, the other from an obscure variety of strophanthus seed. Analysis quickly eliminated the first substance.

Then Reichstein began searching for the second steroid, which was supposed to be found in one of the many strains of strophanthus, some 35 of them growing in Africa alone. The commercially available *Strophanthus hispidus* turned out to be a blank. (See also page 176 ff.)

Reichstein examined all supplies of strophanthus seed that he could get his hands on. As already mentioned, strophanthus seed was a commercial commodity used in the preparation of heart injections. One day, in an old pharmacy in Zofingen—which, by the way, still exists—he came across 100 g of strophanthus seed, mistakenly identified as *Strophanthus hispidus.* He examined the seed. Miraculously, it yielded the world's first and only steroid carrying an oxygen atom at C-11. However, from what parent plant had this obviously mislabeled seed come? Reichstein wanted to outfit an expedition to Africa to search for the seed that would make large-scale production of corticoids possible, but the war broke out and put an end to his plans.

Finally, in 1947, the expedition got under way. Two of Reichstein's assistants traveled across the Gold Coast, Togo, the Ivory Coast and Nigeria. They collected numerous samples, but none of them contained the steroid found in the Zofingen pharmacy. Subsequent attempts to obtain supplies of seed were foiled by outrageous prices and time-consuming negotiations with dealers who could scent a lucrative transaction. Reichstein became annoyed, and the investigation ceased.

About those years and the 1950 Nobel Prize, Reichstein talks with great self-irony. He would much rather reminisce about his childhood in Poland, the imposing pontoon bridge across the river, and the revolution of 1905 that prompted his father to send him to Switzerland. While talking about his mother, who had to take in boarders to earn a living in Zurich, melancholy fills his eyes, at the same time reflecting his profound understanding of human frailties. In his youth, Reichstein traveled to Java, then returned and earned his living by performing secret analyses for the chemical industry, an activity he was not to reveal to anyone at the University. "Industry is not the exploiter it is frequently made out to be," he comments, his pleasant Eastern European accent breaking through. Like many other great men, Reichstein disproves the myth of having been destined from the cradle to achieve a certain goal which, guided by a kind of homing instinct, was pursued against all odds. As a boy, he had wanted to become an engineer. Then, three days before his first undergraduate classes, he switched to chemistry. He would never have investigated the adrenocortical hormones if he had known that they were steroids—he wanted to steer clear of Ruzicka's preserve. Actually, he chose them as a matter of convenience. His secret ambition had really been to synthesize the aroma of coffee, and he conveys the impression that this would have filled him with a greater sense of accomplishment than all the hormones put together.

Yet, once involved with steroids because of circumstance, Reichstein became hooked. They haunted him as they haunted Butenandt. Or was it the other way around; was he unconsciously motivated to pursue them? This is not inconceivable since, after working with the arrow poisons and the adrenocortical hormones, he one day came across the protective hormones of grasshoppers and butterflies and, again, found steroids. As mentioned before, his hobby is the study of ferns, but he cannot resist an occasional urge to analyse their roots, which just might contain a new substance. . . .

Isolation and *constitutional* elucidation of the adrenocortical hormones was followed by investigation of their *pharmacological* properties. It was demonstrated that some of these hormones are responsible for the control of glucose metabolism and others for regulation of plasma electrolytes, particularly sodium and potassium. Between these extremes are those steroids whose main function consists in monitoring protein and fat metabolism, the supply of nutrients to the skin, or gastric secretions. However, a clear-cut separation of their properties turned out to be impossible. The consequent problems in terms of therapeutic application will be discussed at a later point.

The functional separation of the individual steroids according to certain, specific effects resulted in an unforeseen advantage to the chemist. Based on the knowledge that all corticoids possess 21 carbon atoms, at least three oxygen atoms, and one double bond, it was now possible to focus on their differences and, suddenly, it became quite clear that there was a definite relationship between the specific biological *activity* and the *structure* of a given steroid molecule.

Figures 3–41 through 3–43 show that the gradual addition of hydroxyl groups at C-11 and C-17, changes the properties of these substances;

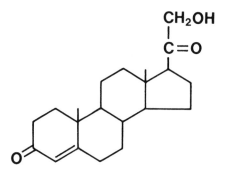

Fig. 3–41. Cortexone (desoxycorticosterone).

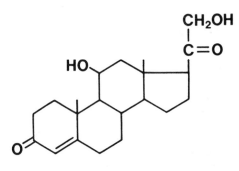

Fig. 3–42. Corticosterone.

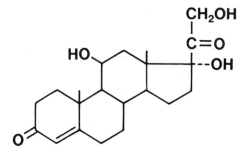

Fig. 3–43. Cortisol.

cortexone (with no hydroxyl groups) has the greatest influence on mineral metabolism—it is a "mineralocorticoid;" corticosterone (with one hydroxyl group at C-11) manifests activity that is somewhere between the two; cortisol (with one hydroxyl group each at C-11 and C-17) is the hormone of glucose metabolism—the "gluco-corticoid" *par excellence.*

In Addison's disease, which is caused by destruction of the entire adrenal cortex, it became possible to attribute the various symptoms directly to deficiencies of individual hormones. Addison's disease represented the negative image of the adrenocortical hormone mosaic. Conversely, this knowledge yielded the key to understanding a disease, described in 1930 by neurologist Harvey Cushing, and attributed to a hypophyseal tumor. Cushing's patients suffered from weight gain, muscular weakness, and swellings of face and neck, referred to as moon face and buffalo-hump, symptoms that are similar to the manifestations of *overmedication* with corticoids.

The next question was obvious. What was the connection between the hypophysis and the adrenal cortex? Investigation revealed a regulatory mechanism similar to the ones we already know from vitamin D and the sex hormones: when needed, the *control* hormone is produced (or overproduced, as in Cushing's disease) in the hypophysis. It is called ACTH (adrenocorticotropic hormone) and stimulates the adrenal cortex to produce corticoids. Corticoid production is measured by the so-called hypothalamus, a basal brain region, in which feedback of adrenocortical activity is coordinated with input signalling corticoid requirements that may exist in various body tissues. When blood levels of corticoids are adequate, the hypothalamus decreases the amount of CRF (corticotropin-releasing factor) released, whereupon the hypophysis reduces secretion of ACTH and, in turn, corticoid production is cut back as well. Figure 3–44 illustrates the principle of this mechanism. In Cushing's disease, the hypophyseal tumor simply secretes too much ACTH and thereby causes an *overproduction* in the adrenal cortex.

To sum up, the effects of deficient as well as excessive functioning of the body's most complicated gland had been recognized, defined and ascribed to *specific* hormones. The logical question arising from this accumulation of information was how one might integrate the overall function of the adrenal cortex within a unifying concept such as that embodied in the key word "reproduction" for the sex hormones, or "cell membrane" for cholesterol. Did the corticoids actually serve a unified purpose, or were they merely a random collection of diverse hormones whose production in a single gland was determined by economical factors? The answer was to come from a young Hungarian who solved the problem by approaching, like Addison, not from the organ but from the manifestations of disease.

In 1842, an English physician, Curling, had observed that patients who had sustained severe burns developed ulcers. Twenty years later, Billroth in

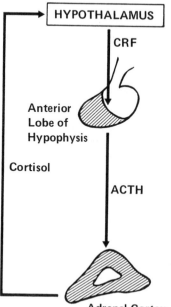

Fig. 3–44. Regulatory mechanism for cortisol.

Vienna noted similar symptoms in those of his surgical patients whose recovery involved complications. Other clinicians reported heart attacks following excitement or exertion, or else emaciation and listlessness as an aftermath of recovery from serious illness.

It must have been around 1926 when a young Hungarian medical student, Hans Selye, began wondering why patients suffering from different diseases regularly developed complications that had *nothing* whatsoever to do with the original illnesses while, *from patient to patient,* these symptoms were peculiarly alike. Again and again, he observed gastrointestinal syndromes, weight loss and depression. He considered these nonspecific features of disease to be expressions of a primordial condition of "being sick" and tried in vain to define the general symptoms in measurable terms. For a long time, he could not come up with an answer, but he did not forget the problem. It took 10 years before he saw an opportunity to answer his question. In 1936, when Selye injected rats with various organ extracts to examine them for hormonal activity, he found to his surprise that, despite the differences in the injected substances, certain common symptoms developed: enlarged adrenal cortices, shrinkage of the thymus gland and lymph nodes, and, again, gastrointestinal symptoms similar to those his human patients had exhibited 10 years earlier. (Fig. 3–45.)

Selye recalled the burn victims with ulcers, the surgery patients with severe loss of appetite, the tuberculars with depressions. Had he finally discovered the pure symptoms of "disease as such," independent of the initial cause? Or did his rats simply exhibit a reaction to the gland extracts? To make sure, he repeated his experiments, this time traumatizing the animals by subjecting them to extreme cold, heat or infections. Over and over again, in spite of the differences between the types of "noxious agents" applied, he noted the same enlarged adrenals and concomitant aforementioned reactions of a body attempting to fight diverse kinds of damage by monotonously always resorting to the same defensive strategy.

In a paper he published on this strange finding, Selye named this reaction the "general adaptation syndrome" or, simply, the "stress syndrome." The concept of stress, practically a household word today, includes the classic sequence of *alarm* (when the body, almost succumbing to attack, desperately mobilizes all its resources), the stage of *resistance* (when the mobilized resources hold back the attack), and the stage of *exhaustion* (when, in case of continued exposure, the body's resources are exhausted and breakdown ensues). Selye questioned the purpose of this nonspecific stress syndrome that has absolutely no connection with the injury which elicits it. The body *does* have a repertory of very specific responses to particular kinds of damage: swelling of nasal membranes against hay fever pollen, inflammation of the skin in case of burns, abscess from infections, or regeneration of blood corpuscles after severe hemorrhage. Why, over and above these responses, is there always this nonspecific reaction?

Selye came to the conclusion that the stress syndrome represents the body's attempt to restore its internal equilibrium which has been disturbed by the specific individual response measure. This is especially true when the specific response (as, for instance, in hay fever) is exaggerated and has adverse effects on the rest of the body, or when (as in serious illnesses) it is basically justified but, on the whole, threatens to become unbearable to the patient. As had been known since antiquity, the body, as an integral unit, can function well only if all its parts are in a state of harmonious balance. The ancient Greeks had called it homeostasis, and Claude Bernard spoke of the *milieu intérieur*. According to Selye, the adaptation syndrome is the manifestation of the body's natural effort to maintain this homeostasis, this balance. Or, rather, it is actually an indication that this harmonizing effort has been overtaxed, eliciting always the same stereotyped rhythm of the "symptoms of illness-in-general"–alarm, resistance, exhaustion.

Just what is the connection between this concept of stress and the adrenal glands? Well, there was *one* clear-cut symptom that was evidence of a relationship: the massive supply of blood to the adrenals which Selye observed after severe trauma. Once this relationship had been recognized, it was soon established that in this nonspecific defense reaction of the body, the glucocorticoids play a major, if not the most important role. Above all, they inhibit exaggerated specific reactions of individual tissues for the benefit of the body as a whole. Simultaneously, through their influence on metabolism, they provide the organism with the energy required for defense against the injury and maintain the blood pressure at the necessary level. An exaggeration of this activity is sometimes encountered in therapy, when very large amounts of corticoids must be administered and, consequently, the patient develops ulcers, muscle wasting, and depression–symptoms that are indicative of "disease as such."

Based on these unambiguous findings, it is the generally accepted view today that the function of the glucocorticoids consists in maintenance of homeostasis under stress-producing conditions. Consequently, their importance is equivalent to that of the hormones controlling reproduction, defense and salt regulation.

Today, because of the connection between corticoids and stress, a great deal of attention has been focused on these hormones. Yet, while any high school student knows about the relationship between distress and ulcers, or excitement and heart attack, errors have crept in along with popularization of the stress concept. We speak of stress and are referring to the stress-

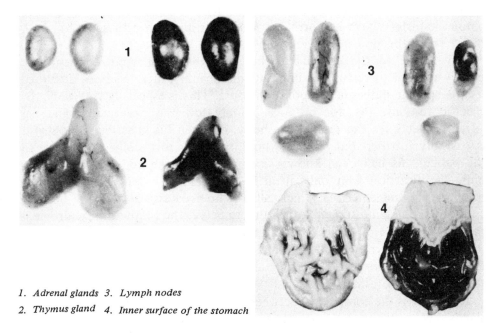

1. *Adrenal glands* 3. *Lymph nodes*
2. *Thymus gland* 4. *Inner surface of the stomach*

Fig. 3-45. Stress reactions in the rat. Left: normal organs; right: organs exhibiting stress reactions.

producing agent rather than our body's reaction; we equate stress and nervous exhaustion, despite the fact that stress reactions are observable in animals that have no nervous system. However, the greatest misconception probably resides in the belief that stress is produced only by disagreeable influences and that it must be avoided.

Selye, more than anyone else, has been emphasizing the fact that stress is part of life. To prove it, at age 68, he gets up at five o'clock every morning to jog, before subjecting himself to additional stressors at his institute in Montreal, which last until six o'clock at night. Stress, to Selye, is life, and life is stress. His enthusiasm has not abated in 30 years; he is equally ready to participate in a discussion on modern child rearing practices and a symposium on the extrarenal effects of aldosterone. He has 28 books to his credit, as well as more than 1400 published papers. He earned 3 doctorates, received 16 honorary doctoral degrees, and is presently busy writing yet another book. Not only is Selye a man who generates his own enthusiasm, but he is also able to instill enthusiasm in others. This capacity was the stimulus, many years ago, that eventually led (through an erroneous assumption) to the therapeutic application of the glucocorticoid hormones. After the glucocorticoids had been successfully isolated, scientists were initially

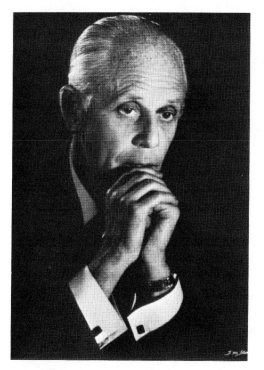

Fig. 3–46. Hans Selye.

at a loss as to their usefulness. Since human adrenal cortices usually function quite satisfactorily, there seemed to be no point to this type of therapy.

During the 10-year span between 1930 and 1940, there was hardly a serious researcher who would have considered clinical use of corticoids— least of all in connection with a chronic disease wuch as rheumatoid arthritis. "The most untractable, obstinate, and crippling disease that can befall the human body," it had been called, "and by its cases of ruin and despair, in one sense more malignant than cancer." What possible link could exist between this disorder of the connective tissue and the hormones of carbo- hydrate and protein metabolism? To understand the connection, it is necessary to go back a long way. As with other refractory diseases, occasional cases of spontaneous remission of rheumatoid arthritis had received a great deal of attention, beginning in the nineteenth century, in hopes that they might provide a clue to therapy. However, these cases were so rare and so unpredictable that an air of therapeutic pessimism soon began to spread, which extended well into the present century. All the more impressed was young Dr. Philip S. Hench at the Mayo Clinic when, on April 1, 1929, an elderly patient reported that the pain in his joints had suddenly disappeared

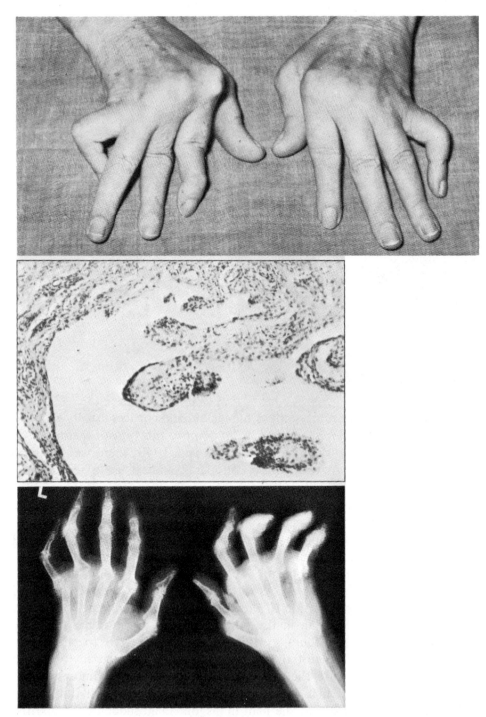

Figs. 3–47, 3–48 and 3–49. Advanced rheumatoid arthritis. Center: inner layer of perio-steum.

after a spell of jaundice. Over the following five years, Hench observed a additional 16 cases of rheumatoid patients developing jaundice. He found temporary amelioration whenever the blood contained a certain amount of bile. Other clinicians began to pay attention and were able to confirm a correlation.

The mysterious substance that might be causing remission gave rise to much futile speculation. Bile salts as well as bile pigments were prescribed for some rheumatoid patients, while others were given liver extracts or injections of blood from jaundiced patients, but to no avail. One despondent patient even had jaundice artifically induced—hemolytic anemia was the result. Failure of all these measures directed the attention of clinical investigators to a hypothetical substance which might have nothing to do with the liver, but was presumedly produced as a protective agent in cases of jaundice. It was named "substance X."

The assumption that this might be a nonspecific protective agent was supported by incidental observations of slight symptomatic relief during pregnancy. In 1931, Hench started collecting relevant case histories, suspecting for the first time the existence of a common ameliorating factor which appeared in jaundice as well as pregnancy. In 1938, he wrote: "It is not illogical to suppose that the agents responsible for both these phenomena are closely related, perhaps identical." He continued with a very interesting comment whose significance becomes evident only in retrospect: "It is interesting to note the close chemical relationship between cholesterol [which may increase in blood in both jaundice and pregnancy], vitamin D [used in rheumatoid therapy at the time], and some of the sex hormones [likewise used in therapy], as well as cortin and the bile acids."

Even though he mentions cortin, Hench's subsequent speculations do not include the hormones of the adrenal cortex. On the other hand, he rules out the notion that the hypothetical antirheumatic agent might be a sex hormone, since men and women alike benefit from jaundice. In addition, improvements were not correlated with plasma hormone levels, and treatments using testosterone and female hormones had produced no striking results.

Then it was discovered, that the hypothetical nonspecific substance was apparently effective not only against rheumatoid arthritis but also against allergies, such as hay fever, asthma or sensitivity to egg whites. While the circle of diseases amenable to improvement by "factor X" was widening, the years from 1938 to 1948 were a period of countless conferences in Rochester between Hench and Kendall, to discuss the identity of the mysterious "substance X." They had no inkling that it was being isolated but a few yards away; it was the compound E on which Kendall's research group had been working in cooperation with Reichstein in Switzerland. In one instance, in

January, 1941, Kendall mentioned that compound E had been found to increase resistance to typhoid infections in mice. Hench recorded this fact as remarkable in his pocket notebook; however, since the amounts available were insufficient for testing in humans, the logical next step could not be taken at the time.

Meanwhile, additional circumstances were revealed which brought spontaneous relief to rheumatoid patients, such as typhoid vaccination, surgery and short-term starvation. More and more voices thus became audible, suggesting a link with the adrenal gland, because all the aforementioned conditions (including jaundice and pregnancy) that had been followed by symptomatic remission were exactly those in which Selye had observed the manifestations of the stress syndrome. Since, according to Selye's concept, the secretion of corticoids represented a specific response to nonspecific stress-producing agents, it was speculated that these hormones might have a beneficial effect in cases of rheumatoid arthritis.

Hench became preoccupied with the notion that rheumatoid patients were suffering from adrenocortical insufficiency. However, no one could foresee in 1941, let alone in 1938, that the substance he was looking for was Kendall's compound E. Years went by and, in accordance with the plan established during the war years, chemists concentrated their initial efforts on compound A. By March of 1945, it had been isolated. In the meantime, clinical investigators had become disenchanted with the dallying of the chemists. When it turned out that compound A had no greater effect on the mineral metabolism of patients with Addison's disease than corticosterone, which had been discovered in 1937, and, furthermore, did nothing to alleviate the concomitant weakness and depression, clinicians were quick to shelve the substance. They had been fed up ever since the experience with DOCA, synthesized in 1937 by Reichstein (which we will learn more about in Chapter 4). That substance had so thoroughly prevented sodium deficiencies in Addison's disease that some patients, prematurely treated because of a wave of irresponsible sensation mongering, had died of salt retention.

In the wake of these events, clinicians awaited further offerings of the chemists, but their patience was running out. By April of 1948, when Kendall had finally succeeded in isolating compound E, practically no one was interested. The long chain linking one disappointment to another, had worn down the enthusiasm of even the loftiest idealists. For Kendall, it was the worst letdown of his life when there was no one willing to test this substance on which he had worked for 18 years. However, Hench, who had not forgotten Kendall's observation in 1941, soon found out that a few grams of a new adrenocortical hormone were available which no one wanted. It was difficult to get in touch with Kendall who, deeply disappointed, had gone into seclusion in his remote log cabin, but Hench was not easily discouraged. Early in

September, through a farmer's old-fashioned telephone, he was able to ferret out his friend and claim the entire amount of compound E for his rheumatoid patients. Kendall agreed, and together they determined, rather at random, that the daily dose per patient should be 100 mg, by far exceeding the daily output of the adrenal cortex, as was discovered later on. In this way, the mistaken assumption that arthritic patients suffer from adrenal insufficiency, combined with an erroneous estimate of the amount of hormone deficiency, resulted in one of the luckiest winning shots in the history of medicine.

Prior to clinical testing, it was necessary to convince Merck to hand over their entire supply of compound E which, under Kendall's direction, had taken years to accumulate. They were generous; all that was asked of Hench was a medical justification, which he quickly supplied. One gram of the precious substance was delivered to St. Mary's Hospital in Rochester where Hench was chief of the Rheumatology Department. On September 21, 1948, the first dose of 100 mg of compound E was given by intramuscular injection to "Mrs. G." who had declared her willingness to undergo any kind of treatment if it would only alleviate the pain she was suffering. By September 24, the patient was markedly improved. Hench and Kendall were jittery with tension. On September 27, the pain in her joints and muscles had disappeared almost entirely, and swelling and tenderness of the extremities had diminished considerably. On September 28, for the first time in years, Mrs. G. went downtown to do some shopping—and, for the first time in years, she was without pain.

No one dared shout "Miracle!" After all, *one* patient could be a matter of coincidence. Then, in November, a second patient and, subsequently, a third and fourth were included in the therapeutic test, and observed with awe and apprehension. Again, there was significant improvement. This encouraged Hench and his associates to perform a scientifically designed experiment, complete with placebo and all the trimmings. In mid-December, treatment of patient No. 5 began with six injections of cholesterol—without any noticeable effect. On December 24, without informing the patient, the injection was switched to compound E. The miracle occurred on Christmas Day. The despondent patient, a shipping agent, who had lost interest in everything, got out of bed, took a little walk around, and started to read again.

Dr. Hench was convinced, but now it was necessary to convince the medical profession. Over the following three months, he carried out additional placebo tests with 18 patients, starting with compound E, switching to cholesterol, briefly interrupting treatment, and doing his best to discredit the new hormone. However, each time, therapeutic activity was clearly exhibited by this substance that no one had wanted any part of.

In light of the incidents involving DOCA and, furthermore, because there was not enough compound E available for treatment of additional patients, all parties concerned agreed to absolute secrecy, but to no avail. On April 20, when the most eminent rheumatologists of the United States were invited to attend a conference at the Mayo Clinic, they knew that a new medication had been discovered—a drug that was effective against rheumatoid arthritis, which had previously been considered a more or less relentlessly progressive disease. Just how wrong the leading medical experts of a country can be with regard to new developments was demonstrated by a little experiment that Hench thought up. During a reception at his home, he asked each of his guests to indicate on a slip of paper his assumption on the nature of the new medication. Not a single one mentioned a hormone of the adrenal cortex!

April 20 became a historic day. There was a film presentation of arthritic patients who had been suffering excruciating pain—cripples confined to their wheelchairs. After three days of treatment, they were shown hurdling tables and benches like athletic youngsters. "Only a phlegmatic person," Kendall writes about this day, "can watch that film without a lump in his throat or a mist over his eyes."

The relationship between the corticoids and therapy had finally been established. It was like a miracle, like another penicillin. Newspaper headlines hailed it, books were written, and the excitement culminated in 1950, with the presentation of the Nobel Prize to Kendall, Hench and Reichstein, for discoveries regarding the hormones of the adrenal cortex, their structure and biological effects.

Hench's discovery not only brought relief to 100 million rheumatoid patients all over the world and led to the greatest concentrated effort the pharmaceutical industry has ever experienced, but it is also remarkable from a theoretical point of view. Until then, only two principles had been applied in dealing with active substances produced by the human body: either they were eliminated (as in castration), or they were replaced (as, for instance, in menopause). Hench had tried something quite different; he utilized a hormone as a medicine by administering quantities that do not occur in nature. While the therapeutic daily dose which he injected in cases of rheumatoid arthritis amounted to 100 mg, the human body produces only 20–30 mg per day. That Hench was unaware of this (because the instrumentation for measuring plasma cortisone levels had not yet been developed), and that his therapy was based on an erroneous premise (because he believed that he was dealing with a glandular insufficiency), does not in the least detract from his accomplishment. For the first time, traditional medicine learned that high doses of a hormone will have effects that differ from those of low doses.

This avenue of approach represented such an overwhelming innovation

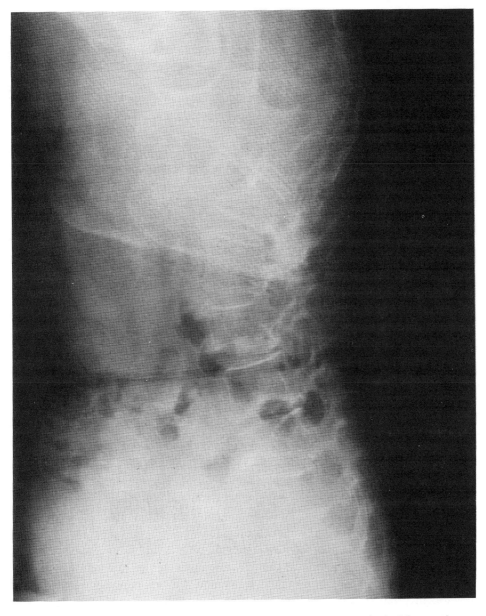

Fig. 3-50. Osteoporosis as a side-effect of corticoid overdosage (spinal fracture).

that high corticoid doses were immediately applied in disorders where, as in rheumatoid arthritis, physicians could not cure the underlying cause but wanted to alleviate the symptoms. Allergies were among the first conditions to be considered for corticoid therapy, because they consisted of a relatively harmless, noxious agent opposed by a massive and injurious bodily reaction, exaggerated out of all proportion. Indeed, the results obtained seemed miraculous. Eczema—which, on the slightest irritation, produced large weeping blotches on the skin—responded; as did asthma and hay fever—which frequently is so annoying that the sufferer is forced to move to escape the pollen. By the same token, allergic reactions to certain drugs lost much of their dreadfulness: edema of the larynx or penicillin shock, which can be fatal, respond to a corticoid injection in a matter of minutes.

We have already spoken of rheumatoid arthritis. Pain and stiffness are not the most alarming symptoms of this affliction. Much more dangerous is the concomitant inflammation of the endocardium, caused by streptococcal infection. In combination with antibiotics, corticoids prevent deformities of the heart valves which can lead to life-threatening cardiac defects.

Then, there is tuberculosis. For years it had been considered too risky to attempt to administer corticoids against this disease, since they simultaneously lower resistance to Koch's bacillus. When chemotherapeutic agents against the tubercle bacillus finally become available, it was possible, at least, to suppress the symptoms of otherwise fatal miliary tuberculosis and cerebral meningitis.

Moreover, organ transplants became a reality thanks to the corticoids. The healthy body, in its striving to defend against any foreign protein, not only mercilessly destroys the implanted replacement organ, but puts itself in extreme danger because of its excessive defense reaction. Corticoid therapy reduces this reaction to a manageable level so that the kidney or heart transplant can function for many years in the host's body.

During those years following Hench's pioneering work, there was finally no ailment left in which corticoids were not used—from tinctures against hair loss to life-saving infusions in cases of shock. It is true that much of this amounted to nothing more than a short-lived fad, but much also has been retained, saved hundreds of thousands from certain death, and made life more easily bearable for millions of others.

We must not neglect to mention the side-effects and risks associated with this kind of therapy. One of the greatest risks is the spread of bacterial infection resulting from diminished resistance. Cataracts and glaucoma may develop in predisposed patients if corticoids are used for a prolonged period of time. In addition, depression and peptic ulcers occasionally occur, as well as, at high dosage, moon face and buffalo-hump which are due to the hormonal activity of the corticoids and have nothing to do with the disease being treated. In serious illnesses such as cancer and certain kidney disorders, the risks or side-effects are knowingly accepted as part of the bargain. In other diseases, the dosage may be reduced, or therapy-free intervals introduced. There are no firm and fast rules since every individual reacts differently. However, this is precisely what constitutes the art of the physician: to steer an optimum course among the advantages and disadvantages, to produce as many beneficial results as possible, and to cause as little damage as possible. Based on this understanding, the corticoids, next to the antibiotics, have become the most important drugs of this century.

CATATOXIC STEROIDS AND ATTACK

There are two possible strategies that the body has available to protect itself against toxic substances. If a rat's paw is injected with a tiny amount of highly irritating croton oil, it will swell, and become reddened and painful. If cortisone is administered at the same time, no inflammation develops; although the oil is not degraded or eliminated, a certain tolerance is built up against it.

This can easily be demonstrated. If, two weeks later, the very same oil is removed from the animal's paw and injected into an untreated rat, extensive inflammation develops—as though nothing had happened before. In the first animal, cortisone merely suppressed the symptoms, without changing the oil's potential pathogenic properties.

The second protective strategy depends on a different mechanism. If a rat is injected with mercury chloride, it will die within a few days from kidney damage. Even cortisone cannot protect it. However, if the rat is pretreated with a steroid called spironolactone, it will survive. If, subsequently, the blood or urine of this animal is injected into a second rat, contrary to the case described above, nothing would happen because the mercury chloride was already destroyed or eliminated by the first animal.

It goes without saying that such a phenomenon had to arouse the attention of someone like Selye, who was already deeply involved in the study of stress. Since toxic is another word for poisonous, he designated the effect of cortisol as *syntoxic* and that of spironolactone as *catatoxic.* The former reduces the reaction and seals the cells against the pathogen; i.e., it is *defensive.* The latter is directed against invaders which it attacks in order to inactivate or eliminate them; it induces secretion of enzymes which destroy the poison or render it water- or bile-soluble to facilitate quick elimination from the body. It is *aggressive.*

The defensive effects of the corticoids had been recognized since 1950, but it took a little longer before the second strategy of hormonal protection was discovered. It all started when Selye observed that the state of anesthesia produced in rats by phenobarbital (or progesterone) is less deep in males than in females. This relative immunity of the male animals disappeared as soon as they were castrated. Something must have protected them (prior to castration) against anesthesia, and it was not difficult to conclude that it was probably testosterone. To test this assumption, methyltestosterone was injected into female as well as into castrated male rats and, lo and behold, their resistance to anesthesia was just as pronounced as that of the intact male animals. Selye, who had already been working with syntoxic steroids, began an in-depth investigation of this newly discovered protective reaction which, as mentioned before, he designated as catatoxic. It is said that Selye and his group tested more than 2000 substances. They discovered that among the steroids, it was indeed possible to identify a group of substances that share this common property. The catatoxic effect of individual steroids varies in degree (and is often aimed against different types of pathogens), but it is unquestionably a clearly definable aspect of their active spectrum. This group includes synthetic substances, such as methyltestosterone, ethyl-estrenol (an estrogen), norbolethone (an anabolic), spironolactone (an aldosterone inhibitor), and PCN (pregnenolone carbonitrile). Apart from testosterone, no specific hormone of this kind has, so far, been found to originate within the body.

From their chemical structure, it is difficult to predict which toxic agents will be susceptible to the catatoxic effects of these steroids. However, for the physician, it is essential to distinguish among poisons against which the catatoxic activity may or may not be effective, in order to enable him to choose the appropriate therapeutic route.

The solution to this problem came from Selye who, in his work with stress, had already started out from the symptom of the disease (rather than from the cause). He invented a system of classification for toxic agents, based on the effect they produce rather than on their chemical structure. Selye divided the "susceptible poisons" into four groups.

The first group consists of poisons that affect the *central nervous system* (CNS), causing symptoms such as anesthesia, spasms and paralysis. It includes progesterone, DOC, tetrazole, mephenesin, and digitoxin in high doses. Against these poisons, he found spironolactone and norbolethone to be particularly effective.

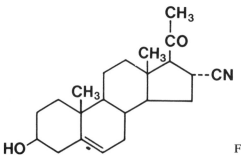

Fig. 3-51. Pregnenolone carbonitrile (PCN).

In this connection, the possibility is being discussed that reactions to other-than chemical attacks might also be channeled into an aggressive direction through catatoxic steroids acting on the CNS level. This means that a threat would be met by counterattack rather than flight. In other words, the question has been raised as to whether there are steroids that can direct an individual's reaction to threat toward either flight or fight. This would, of course, challenge the concept of "freedom of choice," about which any thinking being probably has his doubts anyway.

Some evidence to support this line of thought has already been supplied by testosterone which is supposed to be responsible for aggressive dispositions in male animals. This effect, which had previously been ascribed to testosterone alone, has recently also been observed in corticoids. It has been demonstrated, for instance, that certain steroids will promote aggressive behavior in fish. Possibly, someday, a distinctive catatoxic attack hormone will be discovered, still more specific in its activity than testosterone. Perhaps there are defensive hormones as well: steroids that turn some of us into cowards and others into heroes.

The second important target organ for experimentally induced drug intoxication is the *stomach*. Gastric ulcers caused by indomethacin are the most dramatic and reliable indicators for a catatoxic effect. Rats injected daily with indomethacin, in which each dose is sufficient to cause a fatal ulcer, can be maintained in perfect health for weeks by means of catatoxic steroids. In addition to the steroids already mentioned, progesterone and prednisolone are also effective to a certain degree. On the other hand, there are corticoids that will *cause* gastric ulcers. Prednisolone and progesterone illustrate the fact that the catatoxic effect is not linked to corticoid or sexual properties, but extends across the entire active spectrum of the steroids.

The third symptom of certain toxic reactions is represented by *infarctions*. An infarct is a small area of dead tissue resulting from blockage of an artery. In the heart, it can be experimentally induced by means of toxic agents such as DOC or digitoxin. Likewise, dimethylbenzanthracene, a powerful carcinogen (which we will return to later) can produce similar phenomena in the adrenal glands. Both types of infarctions can be prevented by spironolactone treatment, possibly again through a catatoxic mechanism.

The fourth category of poisons that Selye distinguished, and which may be of the greatest importance from a clinical point of view, has as its target the *connective tissue*. Aging of the connective tissue can, for instance, be accelerated in the rat by high doses of dihydrotachysterol which, in this case, acts as a poison. Hardening of the arteries, inflammation of the heart muscle, and senile changes to the teeth and bones are the symptoms. "Progeria syndrome" is what Selye calls it—we simply refer to it as aging. Again, it can be prevented by steroids, e.g., norbolethone or oxandrolone. The implications arising from prospective prevention of tissue aging are material for a science fiction novel.

Although Selye has defined these four target areas, in which certain poisons are inactivated by steroids, it would be important to the practitioner to know even more specifically against what *toxic* agents this protection is effective on an individual basis. Not all substances which, for instance, cause gastric ulcers are neutralized by the catatoxic steroids. Therefore, it was necessary, besides focusing on the target organs, to define these toxic agents more narrowly according to additional criteria, other than their chemical structure.

Since the "susceptible" toxic agents did not exhibit any commonalities in *chemical* structure, it was attempted to establish *clinical* criteria which would permit a prediction as to vulnerability to catatoxic steroids. The following categories of susceptible toxic agents were defined—the term "toxic agent" applying only under certain conditions.

The first category consists of the fat-soluble vitamins A and D (including the above-mentioned tachysterol) which, because of their low water-solubility, are not readily excreted and, therefore, may cause damage when administered in excessive doses. Detoxification is indeed a problem since, with modern-day preparations, a small bottle frequently contains the equivalent of many liters of cod-liver oil. Accidental or deliberate ("a little more can't hurt") overdosage may lead to serious damage to the eyes and the kidneys, against which there is hardly an effective therapeutic measure other than treatment with catatoxic steroids.

Then we have the many highly potent drugs for heart disease, rheumatism and gout, or sleeping pills, which also produce side-effects in high dosages. All of these respond to steroids. Elimination of toxicity (without loss of activity) would be an eminently valuable advantage since, in these drugs, the difference between effective and toxic doses tends to be so small that occasional overdosage is practically inevitable.

Recreational drugs, such as cocaine or nicotine, are likewise susceptible to detoxification by means of steroids. Possibly, someday, these will permit "enjoyment without regrets."

By far the most important category, which has recently become the subject of increased concern, includes the toxic *heavy metals,* above all, mercury. Years ago, cases of mercury poisoning were reported as curiosities from the mercury mines ". . . somewhere, far away in Turkey. . . ." That has changed drastically ever since mercury has been used increasingly for industrial purposes. Through industrial waste, it finds its way into the ocean and, from there, into fish. Surely we all remember news reports about the poisoning of the entire population of a Japanese town? However, Japan is not the only country faced with this threat. In the United States and Europe, for instance, methyl mercury is used for preservation of seed grain against fungus infestation. This practice is in itself harmless, since the mercury is not absorbed by the emerging seedling. However, if this seed grain (in cases of shortage, or through unscrupulous dealers) is used for animal feed or offered for human consumption, the results may be catastrophic—blindness, paralysis, mental defects and kidney damage may strike an entire geographical region. As yet, we see no end to the potential applications of mercury.

Consequently, there is an increasingly greater need for developing effective treatment methods for cases of poisoning. Selye is one of the investigators who tackled this problem. He injected 30 rats with 0.4 mg of mercury chloride intravenously: 15 of them had been pretreated for four days with a steroid, SC 14266, while 15 control animals received no pretreatment. The control group exhibited fatigue after 48 hours, and all control animals were dead within three days. Severe edema and calcium deposits were found in their kidneys. The pretreated experimental group, on the other hand, was in very good health. To permit examination of their kidneys, they had to be sacrificed: their kidneys were absolutely normal.

Lead is another heavy metal which, as a gasoline additive, is poisoning our air and vegetation (and, consequently, everything we eat) to an increasing degree. Experiments with steroids have demonstrated a prophylactic effect similar to that observed in cases of mercury poisoning. The same is true for cadmium, which is causing severe poisoning in Japan in the form of the itai-itai ("ouch-ouch") disease.

Now, what is the best way of conceptualizing the mechanism of catatoxic activity? In case of the heavy metals, it is possible that the sulfur groups linked to the C-7 atoms of certain steroids convert them to more readily soluble compounds that are quickly eliminated through the kidneys. A similar form of counteraction, i.e., by quick elimination through the gall bladder, has been demonstrated for other medications, so that this appears to be one plausible route. However, for the majority of catatoxic reactions, this is probably not the mediating mechanism. Usually, instead, enzyme synthesis is induced in the liver, where the harmful substances are destroyed. Enzyme activation is specifically aimed at *degradation* of the toxic agent, mostly through oxidation (i.e., by addition of an oxygen atom) or through demethylation (i.e., by removal of a CH_3 group), which frequently reduces toxicity sufficiently.

There are other substances which induce increased hepatic enzyme synthesis. That does not, by any means, make them catatoxic. Insulin-activated glycogen synthesis in the liver, i.e., conversion of sugar into a storage carbohydrate, is an example of a non-catatoxic form of enzyme stimulation.

Catatoxic induction of enzyme activity in the cell is so pronounced that it becomes visible under the microscope. One can see a marked enlargement of the microsomes, i.e., those components of the cell that participate in protein assembly, as well as of the lysosomes which produce the catabolic enzymes. Simultaneously, the rate of cell division in the liver is increased. In some cases, the activity of these microsomes is so intense that the resultant metabolites are deposited within the tubules of the cell's endoplasmic reticulum where they form bulbous inclusions.

As already mentioned, the theory of catatoxic steroids is relatively recent. Almost all the supporting evidence comes from animal experimentation. Even in light of this qualification, the effects that these newly discovered steroids are capable of producing seem like something out of a fairy tale. Yet, it is not too farfetched to draw inferences in regard to humans since, in principle, we possess the same capabilities of enzyme induction as other mammals. We may therefore anticipate that clinical testing will someday yield comparable results.

A certain practical difficulty results from the fact that it takes about three to five days before enzyme induction becomes effective. In other words, the catatoxic steroid must be administered *prior to* exposure to the toxic material. This, in turn, means that if we ever hope to be successful in combating such chronic disorders as lead poisoning or even aging, we must think in terms of continuous prophylactic administration of steroids. Should this be the price our grandchildren someday have to pay for survival, then it will

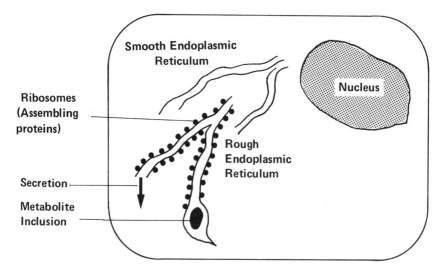

Fig. 3-52. Diagram of an activated cell.

be steep; continuous use of any drug must be preceded by large-scale testing, extending over many years.

As far as instances of acute poisoning are concerned, recent developments are promising. In some cases, the necessary time interval between prophylactic treatment and exposure has been shortened to a few hours. It is, therefore, conceivable that, in the not too distant future, we might take a catatoxic steroid just prior to anticipated exposure to a certain toxic agent. However, we cannot always foresee encounters with harmful substances. Therefore, scientists have been considering alternate avenues of approach, for instance in the treatment of mushroom poisoning, by injecting catatoxic substances into animals for subsequent recovery of the specific enzymes that destroy the poison, similar in concept to the tetanus antitoxin.

While these practical consequences are still a matter of the future, the underlying principles have already revealed two highly significant aspects:

1. It has been shown that the active spectrum of the steroids includes a previously unknown property which no one had anticipated.
2. In the past, hormones had been recognized by their effects or through their absence (Addison's disease, rickets, sexuality) before they were actually discovered as substances. In the case of the catatoxic steroids, it was the other way around: for substances that were already known, it was possible to discover effects that represented an entirely new direction of application.

As viewed from our present perspective, the new stimulus toward additional research activity in the field of steroids appears to be the most important facet of Selye's discovery.

ALDOSTERONE AND WATER BALANCE—THE FOURTH PROBLEM

Life began in the phylogenetic dawn of the Precambrian era—about 1.5 billion years ago. Traces of proteins, a few salts and nucleic acids, which had gathered in the primordial soup to see whether it was possible to generate life on this planet, were confronted, from the very beginning, with a problem whose eventual solution still determines our lives today.

This is because they had to be combined in a cell whose content, to be able to develop such life, had to be different from the surrounding ocean. However, in order to isolate itself from its aqueous environment, the cell needed a wall, a *membrane,* and such a wall creates problems, especially since this was to be a very special membrane. On the one hand it had to allow water to enter the cell with nutrient minerals and leave with waste materials; on the other hand, the concentration and composition of the solutes in the intracellular fluid had to remain different from those in the outside medium, in order to defend the individuality of the cell against the dark and hostile sea. Individuality of the cell included, among other features, a greater number of potassium ions and a smaller number of sodium ions than present in the extracellular environment. It was essential to preserve this disequilibrium.

Two mighty laws of nature opposed this venture. The first is the law of *osmosis.* It is primitive but has awesome power. Applied to this particular instance, it states that, where water can freely penetrate the membrane of a cell, the number of solute particles (electrolytes) must be the same on *both* sides of this membrane. In other words, the total concentration of all solutes in the intracellular water had to be the same as that in the ocean, different though their make-up might be.

The cell accomplished this by evolving a life mechanism that was still functional under those conditions, i.e., where the *total* concentration of ions within the cell, including the potassium ions, corresponded exactly with the *total* concentration of ions in the ocean, with its abundance of sodium. In that way, it had insured its individuality in spite of osmosis. However, the price the cell had to pay was that from the very beginning, all its mechanisms had to be designed around an intracellular particle *concentration* equal to that of ocean water (different though the composition might be).

In this manner, the cell solved the first problem. For its life processes, it accepted concentrational equality with the surrounding sea, maintaining its peculiarity through a qualitative difference in electrolytes. This, however, immediately led to the second problem.

A second law of nature which, like the law of osmosis, is directed toward elimination of inequalities represented an almost greater headache. For example, when a highly concentrated salt solution (perhaps contained in a tea bag) is carefully placed in a tumbler of pure water, according to the law of osmosis, the concentration throughout the vessel will soon be uniform. We already know that. Yet, when a teabag containing a 1% solution of red dye is placed, just as carefully, into a 1% solution of blue dye, the layers will initially remain separate. And why should they mix? Concentrations are equal, and the law of osmosis does not require an exchange of the tiny dye particles. Nevertheless, the next day, the particles will be thoroughly intermingled: the solution will be purple. A process called *diffusion* has taken place.

Thus, nature seeks to equalize not only the concentrations on both sides of a system, but also the distribution of the different particles. This law is effective even when a (relatively permeable) membrane is intercalated, such as represented by the primitive cell wall between the ocean water and the intracellular fluid.

This was a problem that the cell could not solve by resorting to its previous strategy of adapting to the laws of the ocean, i.e., by collecting within, particles equal not only in quantity but also in *quality* to those contained in the surrounding sea. As we already mentioned, it is precisely this which is the essential nature of the cell, that it differs from its environment. This difference means, among other things, more potassium and less sodium inside the cell than in the ocean. Diffusion, however, mandated that potassium exit through the cell wall and that, simultaneously, sodium enter the cell, to equalize the qualitative *differences* between the cell and the sea. Nature does not want differences: mountains erode, valleys fill with sediment, and the earth's heat radiates into a frigid universe. How did the primeval cell solve this problem?

It decided to build a pump that would continuously drive escaping potassium ions back into the cell and penetrating sodium ions back out— both with a force that opposed the natural gradient. This was a highly complicated mechanism which continuously consumed energy. Even today, we still are not sure exactly how it works, but there is no doubt that such a pump actually exists.

Ever since, day and night, millions after millions of year, this sodium pump has been operating in all living cells to insure their survival in the ocean water. This is how the cell solved the *second* problem: it opposed diffusion by means of the sodium pump.

As organisms evolved, for instance into fish, internal channels had to be developed to afford communication between the billions of cells that had gradually formed. These channels were called veins and arteries, the fluid inside them, blood. Within this fluid circulated bodily substances which became more and more essential, the larger the organism and the more complicated its functions. This did not represent a problem for the life mechanism of the primitive cell with its osmotic equilibrium and its sodium pump, so long as the distribution of electrolytes in the blood was the same as in the surrounding ocean to which the cell had already adjusted by its twofold adaptation. This was accomplished by establishing a free exchange of electrolytes at the points of contact between the blood and the sea. While there were primitive, sieve-like filters which were to prevent loss of proteins and cells from the blood *to* the outside, as well as penetration of harmful substances *from* the outside, it was otherwise an open system whose electrolytes were the same on both sides. Its points of contact with the outside were the "primitive intestine" (for ingestion of nutrients) and the "primitive kidney" (for excretion).

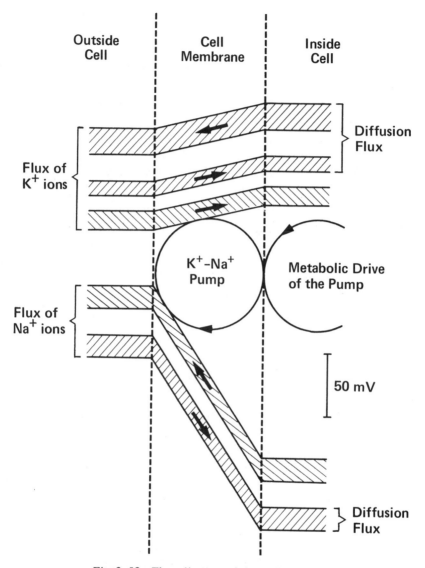

Fig. 3-53. Flow diagram of the sodium pump.

This is how the cell solved its *third* problem: although the organism now had its own blood circulation, the semipermeable kidney permitted the sea to remain in contact with each individual cell which, therefore, could continue operating with its old mechanisms.

Then, however, around 400 million B.C., our ancestors, who had further evolved, decided to go in quest of adventures. What they had in mind was to leave the oceans and migrate up the streams to find new habitats. However, these streams contained a deadly poison—fresh water!

Again, osmosis presented a problem. Fresh water contains few electrolytes, while the cell had adopted a mechanism which corresponded to the primordial soup and its mineral solutes.

What fresh water can do by means of osmosis is demonstrated by a popular experiment for medical students: red blood corpuscles which, actually, are nothing more than "one-celled organisms," are exposed to pure water that, for all practical purposes, is equivalent to stream water and contains no soluble particles or salts. In other words, there is a "forbidden" difference in concentrations. To adapt the intracellular concentration of minerals to that of the surrounding water (i.e., to decrease electrolyte concentration), water rushes into the cells. This occurs with such sudden force that the cells become inflated and eventually may burst. Empty shells are all that is left; these are called "ghosts."

If we assume, for a moment, that primitive creatures had not migrated into the streams but, instead, into the lifeless salt lakes such as exist in the western United States, the opposite would have been their fate. When red blood corpuscles are bathed by a concentrated saline solution, water will diffuse out of the cells to dilute the surrounding hypertonic solution. In this experiment, the pitiable red blood corpuscles shrivel to look like little thorn apples, a condition referred to as "crenated." That is why the salt lakes are destitute of life, and it is also why preserves with a high sugar content possess superior storage qualities: any bacterium, that dares show up there, is immediately dehydrated (see Fig. 3–54).

Now, what were those creatures to do, who found themselves in the domain of fresh water, but were unwilling to give up this new habitat? Fresh water would immediately have penetrated the open-system filters to enter the blood and subsequently the cells, causing them to burst, since they were adjusted to the osmotic pressure of salt water. Those cells that might have survived would have died because of the inappropriate setting of the sodium pump which was unable to change the rhythm it had learned and practiced since the very beginning of life; it would now be pumping sodium out without resistance (idling, so to speak). On the other hand, outside, there would not be any potassium for it to pump in.

Once more, as at the beginning of its life, the cell was facing a decision of great importance. How should it proceed from here? Should it make a clean start and evolve a whole new cell adapted to fresh water? After some experimenting that, no doubt, took several million years, our ancestors found an ingenious solution. Instead of modifying the cell, they invested another

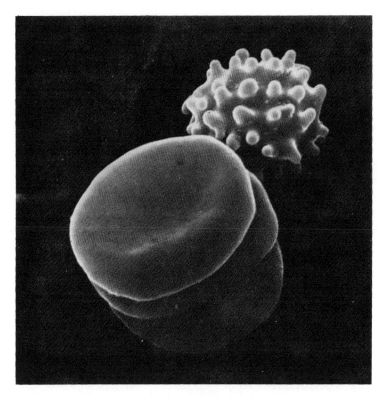

Fig. 3–54. Red blood corpuscles: intact (*left*) and crenated (*right*).

strategy that appears improbable at first glance: they simply took the ocean along on their upstream journey!

They managed to do this in the following way. The two existing points of interaction between the blood and the ocean, the primitive intestine and the primitive kidney, were sealed against the changed osmotic pressure and against the concentration gradient of the salt-free water. Inside, the old ocean could continue to reign. To this end, it was necessary to design a new intestine and a new kidney. Now these two organs no longer permitted indiscriminate movement of electrolytes to both sides, but controlled the flow of the little particles in such a way that the cells continued to be bathed in their accustomed ocean water, even under fluctuating outside conditions. Whenever the cells released too many electrolytes into the blood, causing excessive concentration, the excess had to be excreted by these organs, and vice versa. Using this device, the cells were able to retain the old mechanism of the sodium pump and, at the same time, keep functioning under the conditions they had become accustomed to over a span of more than one billion years.

How can we claim that the blood has retained the characteristics of the primordial soup in terms of electrolyte concentration? Admittedly, we have no samples for comparison. It would seem that there are no clues to be found in our oceans of the present, which have become increasingly more concentrated by leaching out salt from the earth's crust and by the removal of pure water (in the form of polar ice). Or are there?

If we assume (for the sake of argument) that the concentration of minerals in the ocean has, perhaps, increased threefold since the Cambrian period, the *ratios* between the individual salts should, at any rate, be the same in present oceans as in the primeval seas. Based on this premise, the electrolyte concentration of the early oceans should have been roughly one-third of present values. The derived figures for the primitive waters are shown in the following table and compared with the concentrations present in human blood and intracellular water.

Concentration (milliequivalents per liter)

	Sodium	Potassium	Calcium	Chloride	Phosphate
Primordial ocean	141	2	6	165	1
Blood	142	4	5	101	2
Intracellular water	10	160	2	3	100

According to these figures, it turns out that, as far as the most important electrolytes are concerned, our blood is more closely related to the presumed primordial ocean water than to the cells of our own bodies! Even though our premise may not be correct to the last decimal place, the similarity in electrolyte distribution between the blood and the ocean is so striking that we must assume that the blood exhibits the characteristics of the Cambrian waters.

The degree to which various organisms were successful in sealing themselves off against fresh water differs among species. Some creatures, like the herring, never made it and had to remain in salt water. Some pushed ahead as far as the brackish estuary waters where they live in a dilute environment. Others, such as the eel, must return each year to spawn in salt water, to deposit its delicate eggs where they are safe from fresh water. The toughest among these creatures were able to conquer the fresh water of the streams after their kidneys and intestines had been sealed. Those were our ancestors.

Then, one day, some of them crawled on land—initially for trial periods only, like the amphibians. They became the forebears of present-day land animals. However, once again, they had to pay dearly for the advantage gained by mastering a new dimension. This time, the price was water shortage!

The body's own toxic metabolic waste must be flushed out through the kidney filters by means of large volumes of water. From now on, this water was precious. One way of preserving it consisted of reabsorbing it painstakingly after filtration, and recycling it into the blood stream. This task was once again assigned to the kidney which had already performed the greater part of the work during the previous phase. Once more, the kidney was successful. By means of a highly efficient filtering process, it not only collected toxic substances for excretion, but also concentrated the primitive urine 100 times, and was consequently able to return 90% of the water to the body. How did the kidney accomplish this feat?

It simply applied the same principle it had already found useful during the preceding step, i.e., the principle of control of electrolytes. This time, the kidney took advantage of osmosis instead of working against it: the primitive urine and its toxic substances, forced by blood pressure into the nephron, the microscopic filtration unit of the kidney, still contained electrolytes and the precious water. We have already mentioned that the kidney had, meanwhile, gained control over the electrolytes. Now, by reabsorbing only sodium ions into the blood, while collecting toxic substances for excretion, the kidney simultaneously forced the water to abide by the osmotic principle and follow the sodium ions.

The kidney's control over the electrolytes, which serves the dual purpose

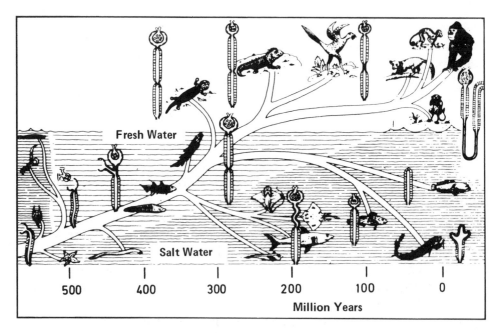

Fig. 3–55. Evolution of the nephron.

of maintaining the so_..te concentration of the primordial ocean and preserving the body's fluid volume, functions by means of the good old sodium pump. Installed on the urine-remote side of the nephron cell, the sodium pump, as in primeval times, forces sodium ions—supposedly penetrating into the cell from the "primordial ocean" (the blood)—back where they belong. What the pump has not noticed is that, this time, the sodium ions did not diffuse into the cell from the primordial sea but from the urine. Consequently, there is an endless sodium migration from the urine into the blood, and the water follows it. Thus, the kidney had solved the *fourth* problem by installing itself (and to a degree, the intestine) as the keeper of the primordial ocean, as well as the body's water balance.

That the sodium pump, while removing sodium, simultaneously loses cellular potassium into the urine, cannot be prevented entirely. This *may* lead to clinical problems when, in case of excessive flow of urine, *too much* sodium is reabsorbed, since the potassium lost in the process is indispensable to the heart cells.

Too little sodium reabsorption, when water is in short supply, may likewise have catastrophic consequences. If the blood volume is reduced too drastically, the body will die in shock unless fluid is quickly replaced.

Like the sodium pumps of other body cells, those of the kidney cells are not endowed with great intelligence. The various occasions that require sometimes increased, sometimes decreased, pumping activity are quite beyond the conceptual capability of a mechanism which, since time immemorial, has done nothing but pump. This brings us back to the hormones.

It had been assumed for a number of years that there is probably a hormone behind the electrolyte-regulatory activity of the kidney: a hormone that controls the body's water and mineral balance (i.e., maintains "homeostasis," as the ancient Greeks called it, or the "equilibrium of juices" which has played such an important role in medicine from medieval to modern times). Alas, however, no one was able to capture this "shy hormone."

The search was complicated by the fact that there were no known symptoms of deficient or excess secretion, as, for instance, exhibited by the sex hormones in castration or, less violently, in the "bearded lady" of the circus side show. This is understandable if we bear in mind that major disturbances in fluid regulation, which in case of shock, for example, are fatal in the matter of minutes, do not lend themselves to extensive clinical observation. The same is true for major changes of electrolyte concentration in the blood.

Or was there, after all, a disease associated with disturbance of the electrolyte balance? Investigation revealed that the lives of patients with Addison's disease could be prolonged by means of a high-sodium (low-potassium) diet, although the symptoms of weakness and fatigue remained unchanged. The more one studied Addison's disease, in which the adrenal glands are gradually destroyed by tuberculosis, the more it appeared that there actually was an associated deficiency of a hormone that regulated mineral and water balance, and simultaneously promoted glycogen storage and well-being.

Consequently, in the twenties, scientists began analyzing the adrenal glands for the presence of such a hormone (see Cortisone and Stress, p. 97). Dogs, whose adrenals had been surgically removed, could be kept alive by treatment with adrenal extracts. Surprisingly, though, various extracts had different effects on the dogs—some were more effective in restoring mineral balance, others in counteracting the muscular weakness and glycogen depletion of the liver. Years went by, and none of the researchers were able to isolate from these crude extracts a hormone that was effective in eliminating all the symptoms simultaneously. There were some who conjectured that there might be several hormones, but the advocates of the single-hormone doctrine were in the majority.

At one point, shortly before World War II, Reichstein produced a steroid that he named desoxycorticosterone (DOC), which was capable of counteracting the salt losses and low blood pressure of patients with Addison's disease. In fact, its potency was such that, administered in high doses, it even produced hypertension and salt retention. However, since DOC was ineffective in combating the weakness and glycogen depletion of the liver associated with this disease, and since investigators were still caught up in the hypothesis that a single hormone could remedy all the symptoms, DOC was not accepted as the controlling factor in mineral metabolism.

A short time later, Kendall found that an amorphous fraction, residual in one of his extracts, contained a substance which was more potent than DOC. When, in 1948, he also discovered cortisone, whose activity proved to be almost exclusively related to carbohydrate metabolism, even the most fanatical adherents of the single-hormone theory had to acknowledge that it was not just one individual hormone, secreted by the adrenal cortex, which controlled the mammal's elementary life processes. The evidence was convincing: there had to be a glucocorticoid as well as a mineralocorticoid hormone.

While the glucocorticoid researchers had realized their objective in the discovery of cortisone, mineralocorticoid investigators made little progress. This might have been due to the fact that one still did not know of any symptoms caused entirely by deficient or excess production of this "shy hormone." In Addison's disease, it was now recognized that both glucocorticoid and mineralocorticoid hormones were absent at the same time. On the other hand, it appeared reasonable to expect that mineral balance and carbohydrate metabolism would be subject to separate control mechanisms in the healthy body, as well as in certain (as yet unidentified) disorders.

Then, an episode from the second World War was recalled, when an American physician, Jerome Conn, had been assigned by his government to find out why American soldiers suffered from exhaustion on arrival in the South Pacific theater. Conn, recognizing a symptomatic similarity with Addison's disease, established that the soldiers' exhaustion was due to excessive salt excretion by perspiration. After a period of time, without much change in the volume of perspiration, there was a drastic reduction in its salt content, correlated with recovery of the stricken servicemen. Conn attributed the exhaustion to deficiency of a hormone which apparently affected not only the kidney and the intestine, but also the skin. This was the first time that the manifestations of a pure deficiency of the "shy hormone" had been observed, but no one recognized the implications. Even Conn, in agreement with the theory prevailing in medical circles, concluded that the resumption of salt regulation was due to the activity of DOC. It sounded logical.

Nevertheless, in light of the accumulated evidence, chemists were still reluctant to accept DOC as *the* mineralocorticoid. They continued to search for a specific, and even stronger, salt-retaining hormone. However, there was a problem. How could they possibly make headway when there was no quick and conclusive test, no bioassay, such as had been developed to determine the physiological activity of vitamin D or the sex hormones, thus leading to their discovery?

By 1952, the time had finally come. In London, James Tait and Sylvia Simpson had developed a method for exact quantitative determination of mineral-metabolic activity: they administered radioactive sodium and potassium to adrenalectomized rats, and subsequently measured the effects of various substances on the excretion of these isotopes in the animals' urine. Using this method, Simpson and Tait tested all kinds of adrenocortical extracts until they eventually found one whose mineral-metabolic activity was even greater than that of a saturated DOC solution. Finally, they seemed to be on the right track. All the greater was their disappointment when a preliminary analysis established the presence of cortisone which was, obviously, nothing new. Such a high degree of mineral-metabolic activity could have been produced by cortisone only if it were present in the extract in extremely high concentration. Tait was therefore baffled when quantitative analysis revealed that the amount of cortisone present could account for only 2% of the effect actually measured. Consequently, this particular extract had to contain yet another active substance. Since this hypothetical substance had, so far, resisted discovery and isolation, Tait was evidently dealing with tiny amounts possessing unheard-of potency. Tension mounted as the promising extract was subjected to fractionation after fractionation, with the activity of each new fraction determined by analysis of the test animals' urine. Finally, Tait and Simpson were actually left with a substance that was 100 times more potent than DOC, previously the most potent known mineralocorticoid. It was tentatively named electrocortin. Now the situation became clear: the extremely low concentration of this hormone had enabled it to elude detection for such a long time. One needed 500 kg of beef adrenals to isolate about 20 mg of this substance. After elucidation of the chemical structure, Tait named it aldosterone. It was the most effective mineralocorticoid and, consequently, of equal standing with cortisone.

Tait and his future wife had only a narrow lead. Results were soon being reported from everywhere: during the same time period, Reichstein's group at the University of Basel, Wettstein at Ciba, the Mayo Clinic, and research workers at Merck had all isolated pure aldosterone. After so many years of searching, the hormone responsible for control of the sodium pump had been discovered by not one, but several independent investigators at about the same time!

The year 1953 represented the first time chemists had discovered a hormone before clinicians had been able to point to a disease that was caused *solely* by an excess or deficiency of this particular substance. Even the suggestions advanced by Conn, regarding the slight deficiencies manifested in the exhaustion exhibited by American military personnel in the tropics, had been worded in such general terms that they had not been interpreted as containing any clues. Thus, the pure symptoms of deficiency or overproduction remained to be discovered.

Again, it was Conn who facilitated the next step. He had made medicine his life's central theme because he was ". . . a little more interested in people than in things." In 1936, when Conn, then 29 years old, had turned to endocrinology, it had ". . . not a very good reputation," as he comments with a mischievous smile. As it turned out, it was this young man from Fall River, Massachusetts, who, with a few others, was to contribute significantly to the respectability of endocrinology, simultaneously ushering in a new era in medicine's approach to high blood pressure.

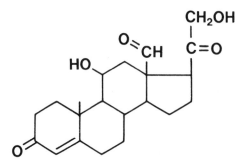

Fig. 3–56. Aldosterone.

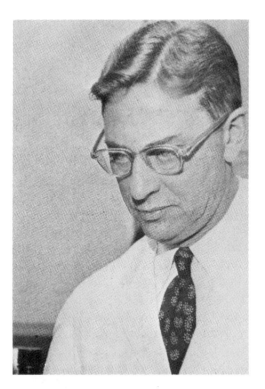

Fig. 3–57. Jerome Conn.

Conn had not forgotten his experiences in the Pacific. If there was such a thing as deficient production, there had to be instances of overproduction as well. He kept on searching, but was unable to come up with anything. One day, 10 years after his first discovery, he was consulted by a patient suffering from inexplicably high blood pressure and excreting excessive amounts of potassium in the urine. This pointed toward excessive transport of sodium in the opposite direction by the sodium pump, and could be attributed to the activity of aldosterone. Since, moreover, this patient and her hypertension represented exactly the opposite of a patient with Addison's disease, Conn was electrified. He thought of his acclimatized soldiers in the Pacific and tested the patient's body sweat: it contained hardly any salt! Here was, indeed, an overproduction of the unknown salt-retaining hormone.

Conn kept the patient under observation for eight months before pronouncing the unprecedented diagnosis of an adrenocortical tumor. Assuming the responsibility for an operation, he accompanied his patient to the operating room. He describes his feelings after the first incision: "Of course, I was looking over the surgeon's shoulder. When, inserting his hand into the left side, he said: 'I can feel a tumor,' I felt the blood rushing to my head and could no longer hold still." At that moment, he knew that he had discovered a disease that had previously been unknown, although it is the underlying cause of 1% of all blood pressure disorders. In his honor, it was named Conn's disease. That was in 1954.

Ever since, an adrenocortical tumor has been the physician's prime suspect, whenever symptoms including hypertension and excess potassium excretion appear. In many cases, this diagnosis can be confirmed prior to surgery by means of contrast-radiography, which clearly shows the swelling (see Fig. 3–58).

Nevertheless, *primary* increase of aldosterone plasma levels represents the rare case of this type of hormone disorder. More frequently, failure of the control mechanism leads to a *secondary* increase; in patients suffering from cardiac defects, kidney disorders or cirrhosis of the liver, part of the serous fluid diffuses from the blood vessels into the tissues (the resultant swelling is called an edema). What initially causes this is not important in the present context. Much more important is the fact that, in this manner, up to 30 l of additional fluid may be retained in the body. Most of us are familiar with the characteristic swellings in the legs and abdomen.

When fluid is thus lost from the vessels to the tissues, certain "receptors" in the blood stream sense a continuous reduction in blood volume without being able to understand the cause. They turn in an alarm, and aldosterone is produced. In order to compensate for the "losses," water is retained in the kidney. In such cases, aldosterone secretion is frequently increased 10 or even 100 times! The more water retained, the greater is the burden on the heart and, consequently, the larger the edema. In other words, it is a *circulus vitiosus,* a vicious circle, which is harmful to the patient instead of helpful. We shall see how this situation can be remedied by another steroid.

Now it becomes a question of how the physician can distinguish between primary and secondary high aldosterone levels, since patients with Conn's disease exhibit increased plasma aldosterone as well. This is a decision of vital importance. Since adrenal surgery would be a mistake in cases of cirrhosis of the liver or cardiac defect, it is essential to establish prior to surgery whether high aldosterone levels represent the primary manifestations of a tumor, or secondary symptoms of some other disorder. The difference is relatively easy to determine.

In order to understand this difference, we must familiarize ourselves with the body's regulatory mechanism for aldosterone. Like all other steroid hormones, the salt-retaining hormone is controlled through chemical, as well as mechanical, receptors and a superordinate protein hormone by means of a feedback cycle. This time, the hypophysis plays a very minor role since the superordinate hormone is produced in the kidney, in the so-called juxtaglomerular apparatus (JGA). In case of fluctuations in blood electrolytes and

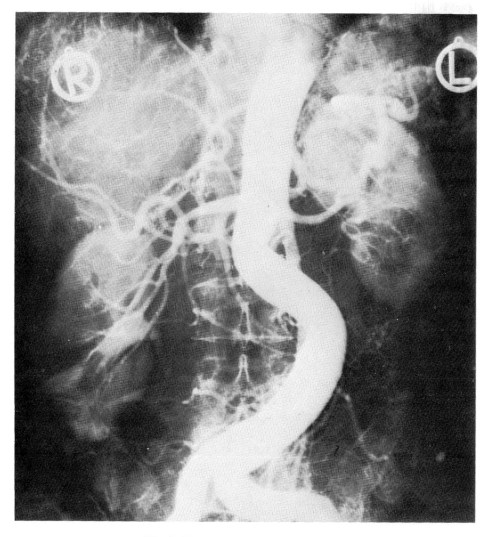

Fig. 3–58. Adrenocortical adenoma.

volume, the JGA reacts by producing a hormone called renin. Renin (via two additional hormones) keeps adrenal synthesis of aldosterone going until the mission-accomplished signal, indicating water and sodium retention, turns off the production of renin (see Fig. 3–59).

Consequently, a secondary increase in aldosterone levels, caused by edema, must be accompanied by simultaneous increase in renin, whereas in case of an adrenocortical tumor, the renin level is obviously not increased. On the contrary—since the tumor produces too much aldosterone in the first place,

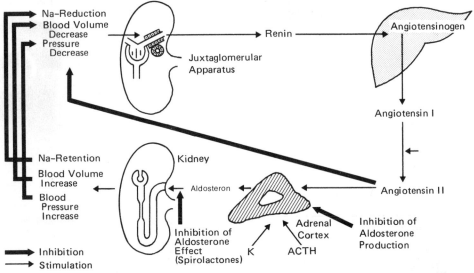

Fig. 3-59. Regulatory mechanism of aldosterone secretion.

no stimulation by renin is necessary and plasma renin levels tend to be low. Therefore, the renin level is the differentiating feature between the two forms of aldosteronism and is used to determine the appropriate course of therapy: in cases of Conn's disease, surgical removal of the tumor; in the much more frequently encountered cardiac and liver disorders, treatment of the underlying cause and simultaneous elimination of the harmful effects of excess aldosterone.

We have already mentioned that this is accomplished by means of another steroid which is similar in structure to aldosterone and blocks the salt-retaining hormone from gaining access to the sodium pumps. We will discuss this in detail at a later point. One fact we should mention here is that the discovery of aldosterone, which initially seemed of merely theoretical interest, has gained tremendous practical importance. Ever since aldosterone's role in the development of edema associated with cardiac, liver and kidney disorders was recognized, and its chemical structure established so that a chemical antagonist could be synthesized, a very large number of patients have benefited. To give an idea of the dimensions of this therapy, it is enough to mention that, in Germany alone, some 80 million tablets of aldosterone inhibitors are prescribed annually.

All this became possible because theoretical conjectures about a hypothetical hormone—whose very effects were unknown—eventually led to its discovery. Thus, aldosterone turned out to be a remarkable illustration of pure and theoretical research, brought to sickbed application within a decade—an example of scientific brilliance converted to daily routine. Among all the steroid hormones, aldosterone has, perhaps, served as the best example of bridging the wide gap between esoteric research and the suffering human being, who alone counts in the final analysis.

4. Surveying the Mountains

How the Steroid Mechanism Was Revealed

EVOLUTIONARY HISTORY OF THE STEROIDS

They come from everywhere—from flower buds and insects, from yeast fungi and bacteria, from fish and fowl, from coral, toads and the tubers of the sweet potato. They are components of the cell membrane, fat metabolizers, cardiac-active poisons, hormones and therapeutic drugs. That is why they are so very important. Without steroids, there would be no life as we know it; without steroids—population explosion; without steroids—pain; without steroids—no love.

They all have the same steroidal skeleton, but differ in the substituents linked to the 17 carbon atoms, or in the direction in which these project into space. In some, the four skeletal rings may have different orientations in relation to one another. This appears to offer little potential for variation. However, the number of possible permutations is astonishing. Thousands of steroids have been found in nature or synthesized by man, and new ones are being discovered every day. It would almost seem as though nature was trying, through this diversity, to cover her tracks.

Yet nature is parsimonious and does not believe in squandering her principles. In spite of this theoretically unrestricted chaos, she has singled out a few groups which catch our eye more readily than all the others. She forgot that this parsimony might put us on her track.

For almost two billion years, the steroids had managed to control life on this earth without putting in an appearance—inconspicuously—quite unlike the sunlight, the rain in the fields, or daily nourishment which acted openly and were easily identifiable as causes of biological processes. Intimately entwined with the principles of life that were accepted as "self-evident," the steroids were thus protected from discovery—by Greek philosophers, by Egyptian and Roman physicians, and by the investigators of the following two millennia as well.

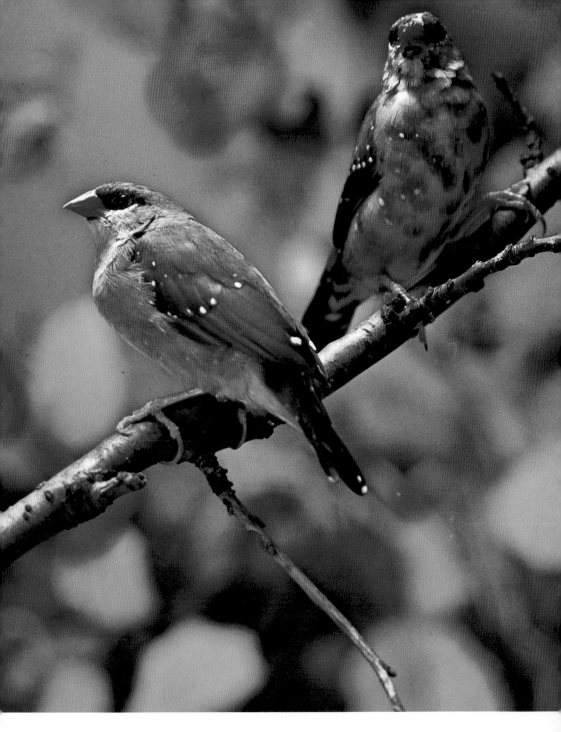

Avadavat pair in nuptial plumage. During most of the year, the male's breast is the color of sand, while during the breeding period, it assumes a colorful brown-and-red pattern.

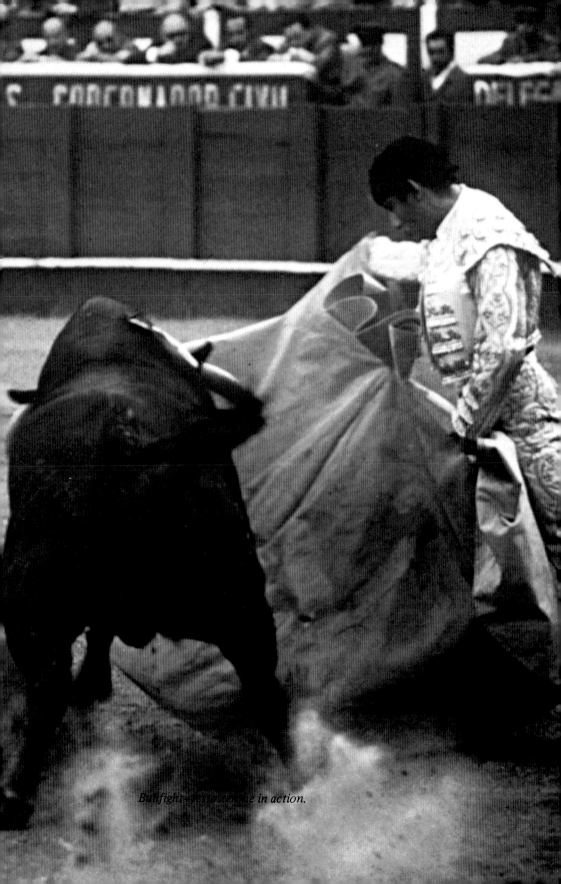

Bullfight—torosterone in action.

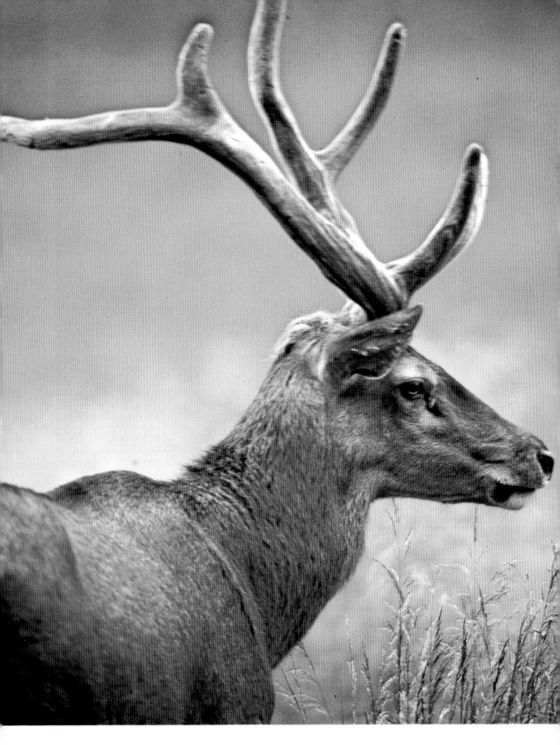

Even the velvet covering the common stag's antlers is under the influence of testosterone.

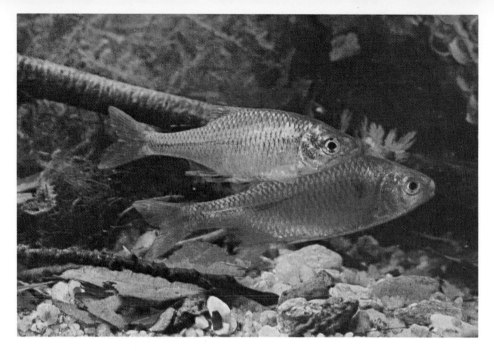

Top: *bitterling. Under the influence of sex hormones, during the breeding period, the male develops a magnificent coat, the female a spawning tube.* Bottom: *a biological mystery—the rainbow wrasse. Through androgens, even its ovaries are converted into testes; females turn into males.*

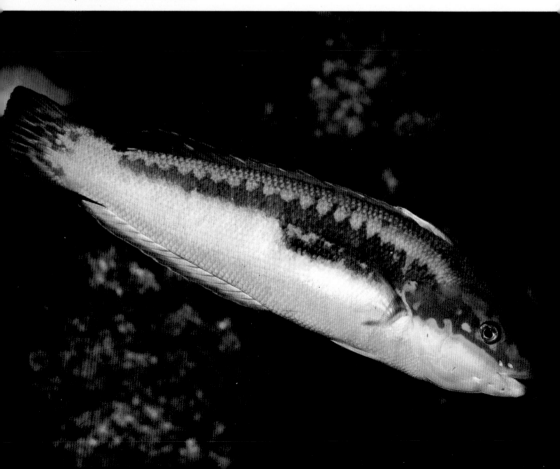

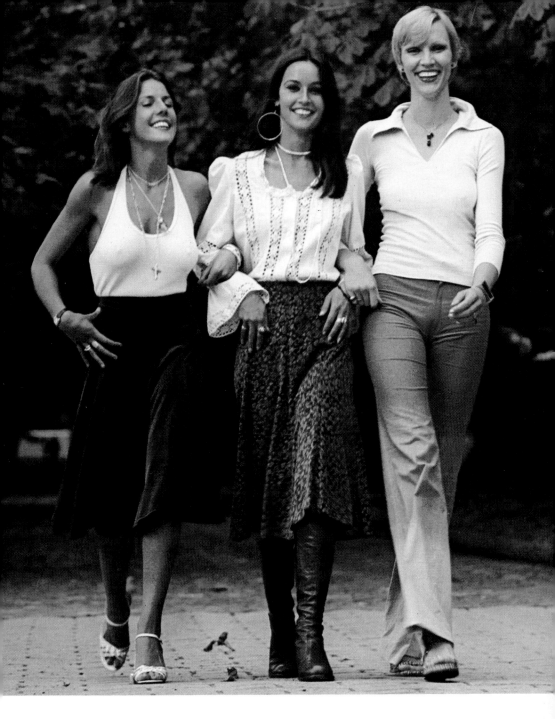

Outward appearance determined by the dominant hormones: balanced type (center), estrogen dominance (left), and gestagen dominance (right).

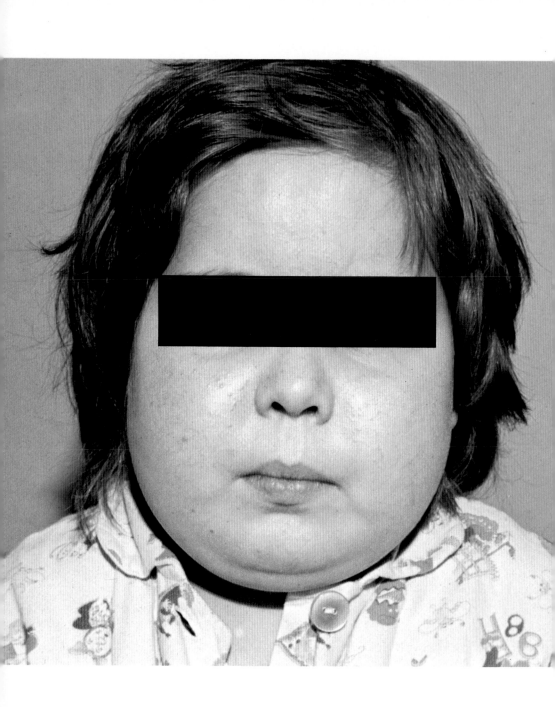

Typical steroid excess—Cushing's disease.

The ocean—origin of all life.
Everything originated from the water!
Everything is maintained by the water!
Ocean, grant us your life everlasting!
Johann Wolfgang Goethe, Faust II

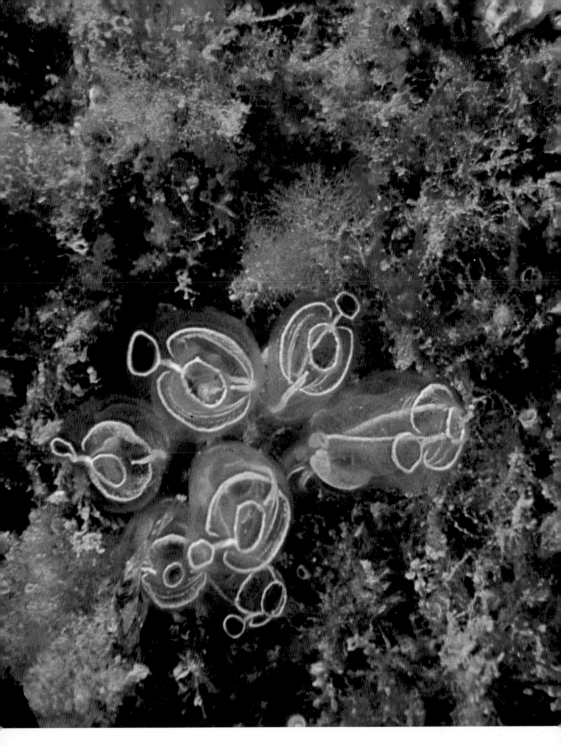

Primitive tunicates—Steroids not yet tied to specific functions.

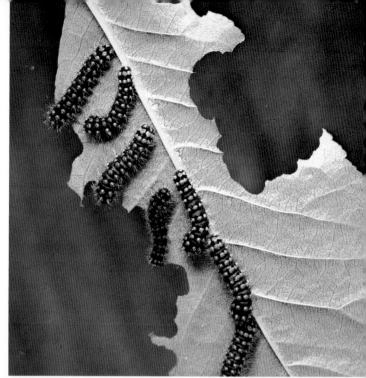

Top: *one of nature's greatest acts,
metamorphosis; influenced by
steroids, the caterpillar goes
through pupation to turn into
the moth.* Bottom: *the moth
has emerged (emperor moth).*

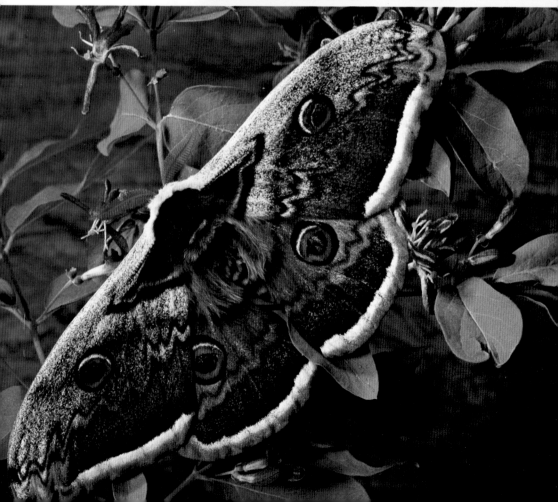

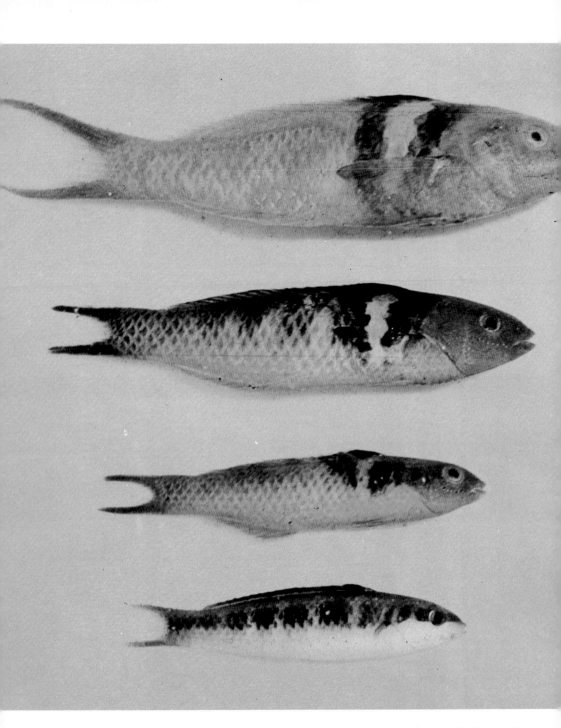

Blueheads. Steroids are responsible for the gradual transformation of the male (bottom) *into a magnificent specimen* (top).

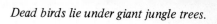

Dead birds lie under giant jungle trees.

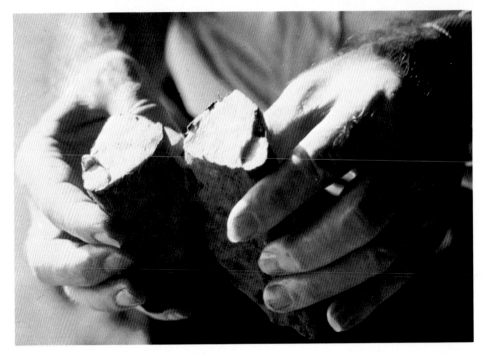

Top: *barbasco root, chock-full of steroids.* Bottom: *barbasco harvest in Mexico.*

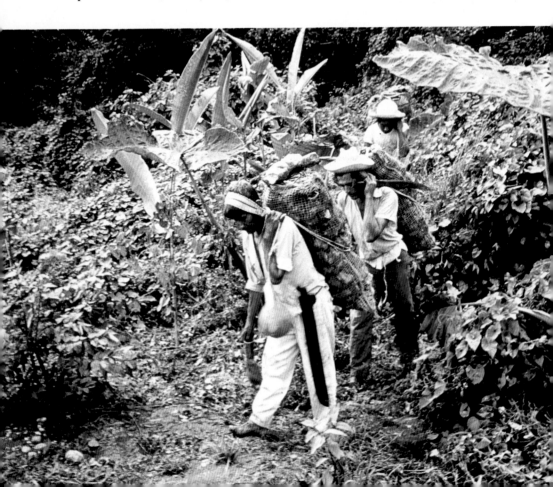

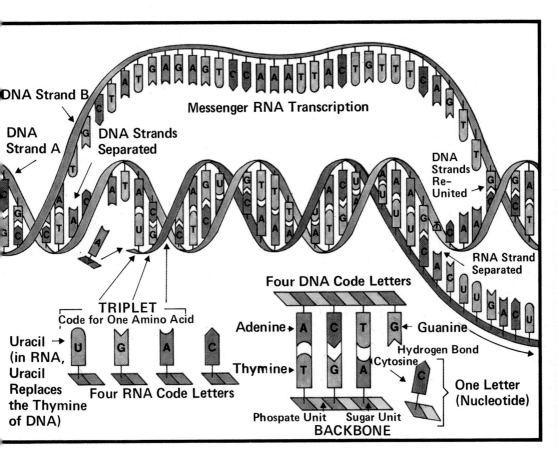

Messenger RNA Transcription

DNA Strand B

DNA Strand A

DNA Strands Separated

DNA Strands Re-United

RNA Strand Separated

TRIPLET
Code for One Amino Acid

Uracil →
(in RNA, Uracil Replaces the Thymine of DNA)

Four RNA Code Letters

Four DNA Code Letters

Adenine → A C T G ← Guanine

Thymine → T G A C ← Cytosine

Hydrogen Bond

One Letter (Nucleotide)

Phospate Unit   Sugar Unit
BACKBONE

Top: *Transcription, i.e., transfer of genetic material from DNA to messenger RNA.* Bottom: *Additions in color show tactical points for improvement of the steroid molecule:* red, *increase in anti-inflammatory effect;* orange—*local effect;* green—*reduced water retention;* blue—*water-solubility.*

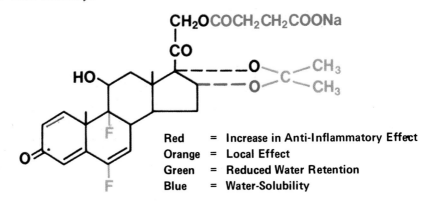

$CH_2OCOCH_2CH_2COONa$

Red = Increase in Anti-Inflammatory Effect
Orange = Local Effect
Green = Reduced Water Retention
Blue = Water-Solubility

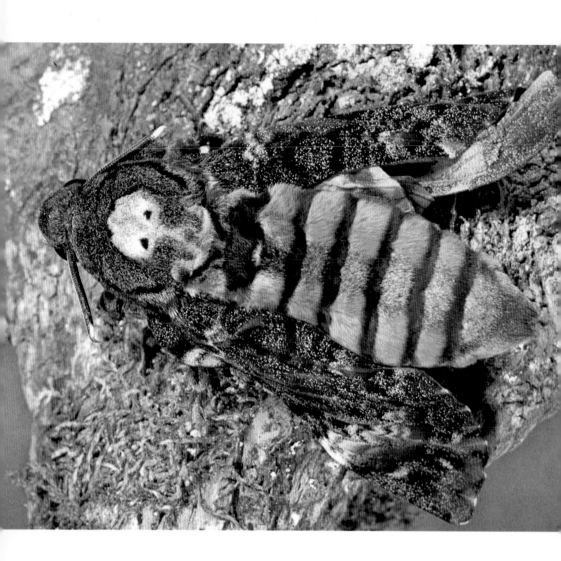

Alternate method of insect control: death's-head moth, deformed by hormones.

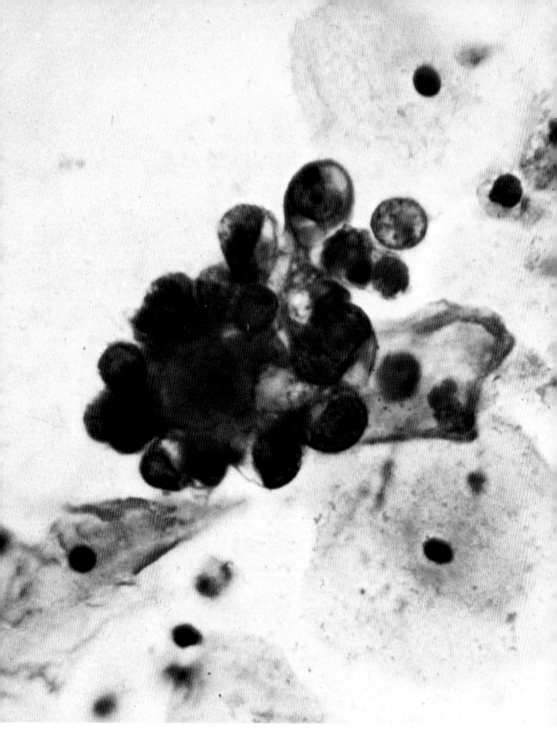

A colony of cancer cells in uterine smear.

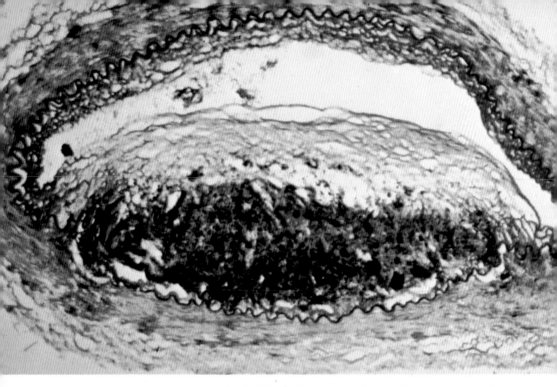

Top: *blood vessel, almost completely blocked by arteriosclerosis.* Bottom: *the first danger signal—two leukemia cells appearing among the red blood corpuscles.*

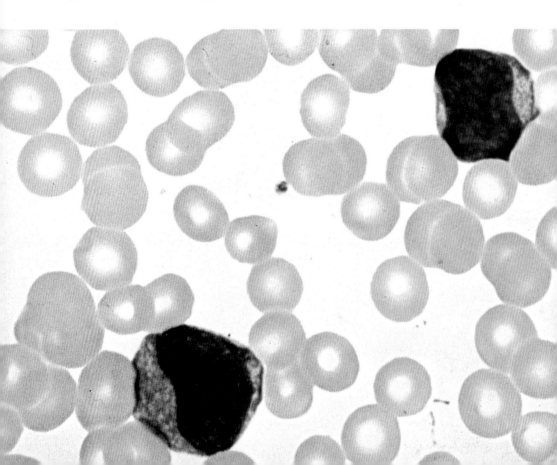

However, the steroids should have known that the puppets they were so artfully manipulating would try to see behind the curtain. We have learned how two initially unrelated events of the nineteenth century were harbingers of their eventual unmasking: the *identification* of the steroids as a distinct class of substances by Chevreul, and Berthold's testes transplant experiments which created the *concept of hormones*. Nevertheless, even at that point, no intelligent steroid had any reason for concern since man was still lacking the tools that could have revealed the connection between these two events. Nineteenth century man was unable to conceive of the infinitesimal order of magnitude applicable to hormone quantities. Moreover, his methods of bio-assay and chemical analysis were pitifully crude in relation to the magnitude of this task. It took almost 100 years to develop the basic prerequisites.

Then, the time finally arrived. We have already reported how, in the golden twenties—unnoticed at first, overshadowed by crises and unemployment—bright spots began to appear; how, in two or three places, the first tiny amounts of potent hormones were recovered, their common steroidal character initially striking no one but the experts.

When, in the forties, more and more compounds of this class appeared, it became obvious that one was on the trail of a principle. Yet its significance remained unclear and resisted all efforts at explanation. Although it had meanwhile become possible to determine, down to the last detail, the features of the steroidal structure, no one could comprehend its significance. It was baffling: Why did nature, so inventive in everything else, work so desperately to come up with ever new variations of the same steroidal skeleton? Why she did not simply utilize some of the innumerable other molecules, of which an unlimited selection was at her fingertips, remained a mystery.

It seemed as though the discoverers of the steroids, having lifted the veil from a previously concealed view, were simply fascinated by the experience without being able to understand its meaning. It is true that scientists soon established the relationship that existed between these new substances and metabolism, reproduction, protection against stress and attack, as well as their role in the cell membrane and in fat transport. Nevertheless, the underlying meaning of the monotonous recurrence of the steroidal skeleton could not be uncovered.

The problem was approached from various avenues, and extensive study eventually revealed a few perculiarities which might shed light on this mystery. There was, for instance, the fact that indications of the activity of steroid hormones were discovered in more and more animals, and even in plants. Where the initial interest had been focused on man, the search expanded, during the fifties and sixties, to encompass life in its entirety. The more organisms zoologists and botanists examined, the more steroids they found. Sometimes they were the same as in man; sometimes they were different. Frequently, the very same molecule was encountered in the alga, in the rat and in man—quite in contrast to proteins, which are different in all living things. However, for the time being, this *cross-sectional* investigation did not seem to lead anywhere.

Consequently, investigators began tracing the evolutionary *history* of the steroids. Perhaps the steroids had evolved from earlier substances, and the details of their development might yield some clues. This was not an organized endeavor. Rather, there were individual scientists who happened to be interested in geological deposits and fossils, and it was only subsequently that the pieces of the puzzle fell into place. The Russians in particular did outstanding detective work in this area. By the most sophisticated analytical methods, they examined all fossil remains they could get their hands on, and each time, they found steroids. Although their sleuthing took them further and further back in time, everything contained steroids. By means of gas chromatography, it was possible to analyze substances from the Tertiary, the Cretaceous, the Jurassic, the Triassic. Further and further into the past they delved, discovering steroids even in fossils from the Permian and Cambrian, the period marked by formation of coal beds. Finally, the last traces ended in the Precambrian—because life had only begun then. The Russian scientists concluded that the first steroids had been biosynthesized by primordial organisms 1.5 billion years ago. However, this realization only served to deepen the mystery.

It would have been a great help to know how, during the evolution of life, the biosynthesis and function of the steroids had changed, and what organisms had been able to live without them. But how were scientists to proceed? How could they look into the past? The steroids found in fossils from various periods of the earth's history were too old, affected by too many changes over time, to provide conclusive evidence.

It was because of a fortunate circumstance that the next step became possible: to find the early forms of steroids, it was not necessary to analyze fossils. Even today, we still have witnesses that have survived from those early evolutionary stages of live. Among them are the oldest of all presently existing forms of life, the bacteria and fungi. Thus, these heretofore despised one-celled organisms became an essential aid to steroid research.

Their ability to synthesize or break down steroids had already been recognized: it was known that yeast fungi synthesize ergosterol and that bacteria degrade bile acids in the intestine. However, this did not by any means imply that they also utilized steroids in their own vital processes. If so, it was perhaps even more important to find out which steroids were involved.

From the very beginning, the work with bacteria and fungi proved to be much more difficult than had been anticipated. First of all, one-celled organisms do not have organs which (like the ovaries or adrenals of the vertebrates) are steroid factories and contain these substances in high concentrations; nor is it possible to collect a bacterium's urine for extraction of steroids. Instead, the whole organism must be processed. This is roughly equivalent to putting 40,000 head of cattle through a meat grinder to extract the 50 mg of hormonal substance which Reichstein had recovered from their adrenal glands.

A second problem was presented by the great variety of steroids found in these primitive beings. Due to their rather nonspecific life processes, various steroids were capable of filling in for one another so that, as yet, no individual hormone had a monopoly. Consequently, no steroid was more essential than the others, as, for example, the corticoids or sex hormones were in man. Moreover, comparative hormone research did not have the same impetus as research which had a direct bearing on man. Research on bacterial hormones is, to the layman, about as interesting as a dissertation on the love life of a June beetle—although its implications are far more relevant to him. Funding, therefore, was limited.

For these reasons, it was not until a few years ago, that it became possible to disprove the hypothesis that bacteria (in contrast to the yeast fungi) cannot biosynthesize steroids. Russian researchers, above all Achrem Affanassi'ev, have established some amazing facts through their research on bacteria.

First of all, based on this research, it is highly improbable that organisms without steroids exist. This is more surprising than it may seem at first glance, for it means, stated in different terms, that there is apparently no life without steroids. Consequently, there must be a commanding force of some kind, that ties the development of life to the steroids. This gave rise to the next question: What constitutes this commanding force? What is it that cannot occur without steroids?

Secondly, these investigations show that even bacteria have a rich pool of steroids, some of which have become extinct while others were retained by higher organisms. Nevertheless, from a chemical point of view, these substances did not undergo further development.

The third and probably most important result of this recent research, however, resides in the understanding that the steroids are generally associated with vital functions and that certain steroids, in the course of evolution, have become tied to specific functions.

It was already known that, in man, reproduction, metabolism, attack and defense, as well as membrane function, are somehow related to the steroids.

It then became necessary to determine the extent to which this applies even to single-celled animals. The enormous difficulties encountered in discovering this have already been mentioned. In addition, we must keep in mind that complicated, coordinated processes do not exist in one-celled organisms. Instead, we find the activities of individual organelles, each serving a single purpose. Nevertheless, it was possible to demonstrate the beginnings of such a relationship between steroids and function in unicellular life. The most clear-cut example is the *cell membrane*: in fungi, ergosterol plays a specific role in the formation of the cell wall. This specificity was retained by plants, while animals switched to cholesterol.

Recently, research workers have succeeded in demonstrating a relationship between the *reproduction* of fungi and steroids: the female fungi of the genus *Achlya* were found to discharge autendiol into the water to initiate sexual reproduction.

The associations between steroids and *stress* are nonspecific: when certain fungi are subjected to stressors, such as heat or radiation, they increase biosynthesis of diverse steroids, similar to the stepped-up secretion of corticoids in man.

The function of *protection* against attack, which we still find in the toad, the sea cucumber and many plants, also exists in single-celled animals. Viridine and other steroids serve to protect bacteria against fungus attack, while, on the other hand, fungi use different steroids as a protection against bacteria. However, the functional specificity appears to be low; in each case, this function is performed by a different steroid.

At any rate, in a unicellular organism, we cannot speak of hormone action as it controls the whole multi-cellular body of the vertebrate. This is because, as already mentioned, metabolism, reproduction and stress, in the one-celled animal, do not require coordination of several organs but merely stimulation of an individual organelle.

If we move up the evolutionary ladder, plants show the first tendency to tie the control of *reproduction* to a limited number of steroids. This becomes necessary because the higher functions are based on complex interactions between several organs. This, in turn, requires that the receptors of these organs agree on one specific steroid to which they will respond for a particular purpose. An examination of buds just prior to blooming reveals a "steroid explosion" in these tissues. Usually, these are of the sapogenin group, the foam-producing steroids. On the other hand, some plants seem to be experimenting with other kinds of hormones. Some of them are the same steroids which the vertebrates have selected as their hormones. Butenandt, in 1930, found estrone in palm kernels; in 1964, French scientists discovered progesterone in *Holorrhena floribunda;* and, most recently, Australian feed plants were found to contain androgens. From the mere presence of steroids, however, it does not necessarily follow that they have anything to do with reproduction. Loew pointed this out in 1945. Looking for an answer to this highly intriguing question, he stirred estrogens into a lanolin paste and spread this mixture on the bud tips of a dioecious melandosum plant which was about to bloom. Amazingly, all the pistillate (female) flowers burst into bloom, while the staminate (male) flowers were suppressed. In a control experiment, he repeated the procedure with testosterone and, this time, it was the pistillate flowers that were suppressed. The initially dioecious plant had been turned into a monoecious one: either male or female, depending on the hormonal influence.

In these plants which, on their own, do not use estrone for maturation, must have resided the memory of other, older steroids that, long ago, had performed this function, but were later replaced by the sapogenins. At the same time, these plants had retained the ability to respond to several substances, an ability that was gradually lost in the animal kingdom. Through this observation, it became apparent that it made no difference which particular steroid took charge of the reproductive function as long as the organs involved had appropriate receptors.

So it seems that there was a period of development during which the plants and animals selected, from the rich steroid pool of primordial organisms, the ones they found most suitable, and tied them to specific functions. We already have some idea as to how this increasingly more rigid association between very specific steroids and particular functions came about. The area of reproduction provides a good example.

We may assume that, originally, the ovaries (or the testes, respectively), the skin, the brain, the urogenital tract, and the mammary glands, each used a different hormone for activation. As evolution progressed, several organs were combined into a target group: the production of ova or gametes was combined with protection of the fertilized ova and competition among males. That meant elaboration of the Müllerian ducts, inclusion of behavioral patterns (courtship behavior), specialization of the skin (tail feathers), and much more. Everything had to be set in motion simultaneously, and that was possible only by agreeing on *one* hormone for coordinating the activities of the appropriate organs.

Basically, it did not matter which steroid was eventually selected for this purpose. There is nothing about the structure of estrone or testosterone that makes them sex-specific; only through the presence of specific receptors in the sexual organs, did they become sex hormones. The basic coordination thus seems to have been implemented through development of appropriate receptors in cells that belong to the same functional group.

The first fixed relationship between steroids and function probably appeared relatively early. Aside from their role with regard to membrane function, it was most likely the female sexual function that first required coordination. In the tunicates, or sea squirts, for instance, none of the steroids stands out among the others. However, in scallops, relatively high amounts of estrone and progesterone very probably mean that these two female steroids are performing specific sex-regulatory functions. In the scallop, the steroids were probably elevated to the rank of hormones for the first time, a fact that we might want to bear in mind whenever we enjoy coquilles St. Jacques.

Subsequently, additional factors of evolutionary significance are incorporated: among the fish with their complicated reproductive procedures, the protective role of the male becomes more and more important. For the first time, testosterone appears fairly regularly and produces aggressive males. Yet, the cell receptors are still uncertain; those of the female animals are not always able to reject the male hormones. This has been demonstrated through some highly interesting experiments that Reinboth performed with blueheads. If the sexually differentiated, but not yet active young males are injected with testosterone, they develop their magnificent nuptial coat and prepare for courtship, as we would expect. In the biologically inactive juvenile females, however, the same treatment will induce the mature animals to convert their ovaries into testes; a process which is no longer possible in more highly developed animals.

Even on this low evolutionary level, the vertebrates already possess an extensive *stress* mechanism which includes control of carbohydrate and electrolyte metabolism. At this point, cortisol and corticosterone become linked to these two functions. Since the reactive mechanism is still relatively primitive, the two steroids remain interchangeable in this case. Only later on, does the former turn toward carbohydrate- and the latter toward mineral-metabolic activity.

To the extent to which animals gradually migrate into the fresh water of streams or venture onto dry land, the regulation of *mineral* metabolism, in many genera, comes under the control of a specific mineralocorticoid, aldosterone.

At this point, the steroid functions have, basically, reached the same scope that applies to man. Not only have the functions since remained the same, but also the steroids themselves. In all mammals, birds, reptiles, and even in amphibians, we find absolutely identical steroid patterns. From polar bear to parrot and turtle, to frog and cod—all have the same testosterone, estrone, progesterone, aldosterone and cortisol.

It is true that some functions which we did not mention, such as defense and catatoxis, may have become lost again, while others might not have developed as yet. However, on the whole, it is amazing how powerful was the force that compelled living organisms to retain the same steroids, selected in the very beginning for various functions, against certainly intense evolutionary pressure: the stability of the steroids from the scallop to man is a miracle.

If we were to draw a family tree of the steroids, it would begin with an array of undifferentiated, nonspecific substances which, during the course of evolution, became concentrated into a few potent hormones that were already present among the original substances. The probability that we are still utilizing steroids from the original pool of the single-celled organism is supported by two remarkable facts. Today's steroids are still being manufactured according to the same blueprint as those of the bacteria: all naturally occurring steroids rotate the plane of polarized light to the *right*. This phenomenon is by no means a matter of course, since those steroids which the chemist synthesizes in his laboratory always result in a mixture of dextrorotatory and levorotatory steroids. Here, it seems, nature is using a stratagem that we are as yet unable to imitate, and no living creature has ever dared deviate from this basic blueprint. The *ingredients* of the recipe have also remained unchanged: biosynthesis of steroids from acetic acid, mevalonic acid and squalene, which we will describe in a subsequent chapter, has been demonstrated for bacteria as well.

All of this leads to the conclusion that the steroids, despite assuming important additional responsibilities, and despite an evolutionary span equivalent to no less than one-third of our planet's existence, have not changed. Herein lies a fundamental difference between the steroid hormones and the protein hormones.

All these insights notwithstanding, we have been unable to take even one little step forward in our search for the reason underlying the unchanging existence of the steroids. Therefore, it might be a good idea to take a closer look at the protein hormones which have gone through clearly traceable changes, step after step up the evolutionary ladder. Perhaps, such a comparison will serve to shed new light on the mystery of the steroids.

STEROIDS AS HORMONAL MESSENGERS

The more the steroids grew into their role as hormones, the more clearly they became differentiated from the remaining hormones. The hormones we have mentioned so far, like parathormone, ACTH, LH and FSH—in addition to their own, generally rather narrow range of activity—are prominent chiefly because of their stimulatory effect on steroid biosynthesis. Of course, there are additional hormones besides these: growth hormone, insulin, the hormone of the thyroid gland, to mention a few. In this select company, the steroids have always remained outsiders, albeit indispensable. The key to understanding them must be to recognize just how the steroids differ from the other hormones.

Adrenaline and thyroxine, the first hormones scientists had been able to isolate, are derivatives of amino acids, those building blocks used to assemble proteins. Later on, when insulin and, in a magnificent series, one hypophyseal hormone after another were discovered, it turned out that they all consist of proteins or their building blocks. Consequently, they all contain nitrogen. Their kinship with the proteins is the first common characteristic of these hormones.

What, at first glance, appears to set them apart, are differences in the sequence and number of their amino acids: some, like the growth hormone of the sheep, consist of several hundred amino acids and have a molecular weight as high as 48,000; others, like angiotensin which influences blood pressure, consist of only eight amino acid units, while still others are derivatives of a single amino acid. Some contain iodine, others sulfur bridges; some are assembled in spirals, others in bizarre formations that resemble hieroglyphic characters. For each purpose, an entirely different molecule was developed. It is precisely this multiformity of the "protein hormones" (as we shall call them for the sake of simplicity) that is their second essential characteristic.

However, protein hormones differ not only within the body of a certain animal, but also between animal species, since almost every species designed its hormones in accordance with its own special requirements. This tremendous variety was created by varying the sequence of amino acids within the long protein chains; sheep growth hormone has little effect, and the bovine variety no effect, on man. This specificity for individual species is the third commonality of the protein hormones.

Let us look at the steroid hormones in comparison. They do not contain nitrogen, and even those which differ widely in their effects still have the same basic steroidal skeleton. Moreover, all vertebrates secrete the same steroid hormones—the cock's testosterone is identical to man's.

Evidently, the breath-taking development from single-celled organisms to man, on the one hand resulted in a great variety of pretein hormones while, on the other hand, it went right past the steroid hormones without being able to either change or replace them. On the contrary, the stubborn steroids have assumed an increasingly more important role. It is not difficult to imagine the great pains evolution had to take in adapting to this unchangeable molecule and developing the diversity of hundreds of thousands of life

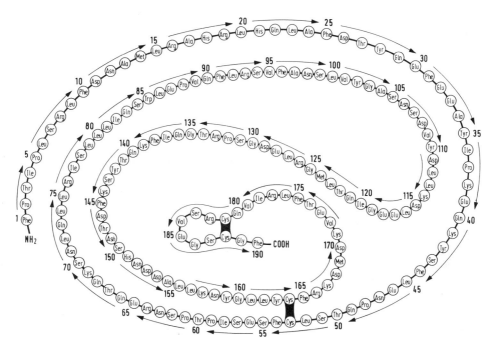

Fig. 4-1. Amino acid sequence of human growth hormone.

forms around it. How many million years must have elapsed before nature succeeded in inducing the same testosterone to cause growth of a comb in the cockerel and growth of a beard in man! Most probably, she initially tried simpler strategies, such as modifying the steroid molecule or utilizing specific hormones, instead of working around the rigid steroidal skeleton. The fact that nature did not succeed in either changing the steroid hormones, or replacing them by the much more flexible protein hormones, serves to illuminate the significance of their role in the evolution of life.

In order to get a grip on the steroid hormones, nature had to resort to a roundabout maneuver: by means of an artful stratagem, she subordinated the steroids to the smoother, more easily influenced protein hormones. How was this possible? In order to be able to understand this, we first have to know something about the protein hormones' functional mechanism which had remained a puzzle for a long time. When it was finally revealed, it was almost disappointingly simple, reminiscent of the anecdote about Columbus and his amazing egg. The Columbus of the protein hormones, who won the Nobel Prize for his discovery, was Earl Sutherland.

What Sutherland established was that all protein hormones influence their target cells in basically the same manner: by binding to a hormone receptor in the cell membrane, they activate an enzyme (adenylate cyclase) which is also present in the membrane and transmits their "message" to always the same "second messenger" (cyclic AMP, also known as cAMP) inside the cell. This, in turn, sets in motion the specific activity that was intended by the hormone and for which this particular cell is specialized. By this mechanism, adrenaline raises the blood sugar level while insulin lowers it, thyroxine steps up metabolism, and secretin increases release of gastric juices.

There was much speculation as to how this mechanism works specifically; how the widely differing "first messenger" protein hormones—although they use absolutely *identical* "second messengers"—finally manage to produce the *diverse* effects that are typical for each "first messenger" hormone. The answer is that the primary hormone can arouse the "second messenger" only in those cells capable of the activity initially intended by the hormone; only those cells contain the *specific* hormone receptor which recognizes "its own" hormone, whereas it will not respond to any of the other hormones in the blood. Via stimulation of adenylate cyclase, the hormone then induces synthesis of (nonspecific) cAMP which in turn stimulates the (specific) activity of that particular cell. This ensures both diversity and specificity. On the one hand, such diverse effects as formation of a corpus luteum or production of milk are coordinated. On the other hand, since the cells of unrelated tissues do not contain this particular hormone receptor, the specificity of the "first messenger" is simultaneously safeguarded.

As Sutherland recognized, the production of steroids is also subject to this simple mechanism; for example, in the adrenal cortex, the cell walls contain a receptor for ACTH. Binding to this receptor, ACTH stimulates adenylate cyclase which in turn promotes (again via cAMP) the production of cortisol. In this manner it was possible, despite the fact that the superordinate hormones were different for different animal species, to retain the same steroids over the entire span of evolution.

The reasons for subordinating the steroids to the protein hormones have already been suggested. To begin with, this arrangement permits a decision-making process based on the various data that influence steroid production. This can only be accomplished by the higher centers: the season and available food supply may call for the onset of mating behavior, and thus for secretion of estrogens, while a sudden threat may prohibit it. Contradictory information of this type must be integrated into one single command that the steroids will be able to understand. In addition, as animals became more highly developed, there was an increased potential for functional conflicts both among steroids, and between steroids and other systems, e.g., in case of excessive amounts of sodium in the diet, where aldosterone (through retention of sodium ions and the corresponding compensatory water retention) may lead to abnormally high blood pressure which is subject to regulation by another hormone.

Conflicts of this nature must be settled by superordinate centers. For complex situations, which occasionally may require a nontypical response, these centers are mostly located in the brain. There, the hypophysis is in charge of manufacturing the protein hormones which convey messages to the glands: ACTH (for glucocorticoids), FSH (for estrogen), and LH (for progesterone and testosterone) are released into the blood circulation in order to stimulate or suppress steroid production. Other centers of a more autonomous nature are located on the periphery: parathormone conveys the message of the parathyroid which collects information regarding calcium metabolism and directs synthesis of 1,25-DHCC (vitamin D_3); the juxtaglomerular apparatus in the nephrons of the kidney, on the other hand, influences blood volume, salt excretion, and blood pressure.

How does the superordinate center find out whether or not "its" steroid has accomplished the intended mission? Well, we have seen how feedback may be provided by direct measurement of the intended result; e.g., the JGA pays no attention to the steroid level but only to the receptors measur-

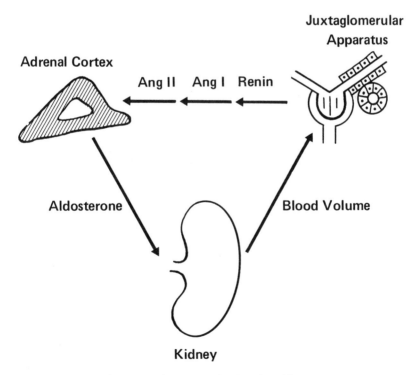

Fig. 4–2. Regulatory mechanism for aldosterone.

ing blood volume: based on their signal, renin secretion is either continued or not. Similarly, with regard to plasma calcium levels, the regulatory mechanism is based on a mission-accomplished signal as well.

However, in most cases, the control center is satisfied with a signal indicating that steroid synthesis is sufficiently high to produce the desired results—without checking whether or not the assigned mission has actually been accomplished. In this case, the hypothalamus, located near the hypophysis in the brain, monitors plasma levels of the most important steroids. As long as readings are unsatisfactory, the hypophysis continues to secrete hormones (e.g., gonadotropins); secretion does not stop until a satisfactory steroid level is measured in the blood.

We have already learned, in connection with contraception, how man interferes with this feedback cycle and takes advantage of it to prevent maturation of the ovum. Nevertheless, we are reviewing this feedback mechanism to illustrate the relationship between protein hormones and steroids. How this cooperative action first developed will probably never be revealed. There is no doubt, however, that the steroids were subordinated to protein hormones that already had some specific, related experience: renin (or angiotensin) had already, on its own, exerted an influence on blood pressure before it learned to stimulate aldosterone synthesis. Similarly, the hypophysis had already performed adaptive functions in the remote past. By influencing the pigment-bearing cells, it caused in fish or frogs, for example, adaptive changes in coloration which enabled them to blend into the environment, perhaps the bottom of a brook. When, in Addison's disease, excessive amounts of ACTH are produced to stimulate the damaged adrenal glands, this old mechanism still breaks through, with fragments of the excess ACTH stimulating the pigment-bearing cells and thus causing the characteristic bronze coloration of the skin. After all this, it should surprise no one, that the sex hormones were subordinated to the gonadotropins (FSH, LH), which influence the germ cells (ovum, sperm).

This immediately brings us back to the old question of why, with all their "experience," the protein hormones even needed subordinates like the steroids whose functions, it would seem, they should have been flexible enough to perform without help. Looking at the chain of events from release of the protein hormone to the final action of the steroid, we realize that the steroid is only an intermediate agent performing a task of the protein hormone. The steroid has become a "third messenger" (see Figs. 4–3 and 4–4), and the question is, Why?

The answer lies in the cAMP mechanism. If we keep in mind that in all body cells, all protein hormones can only activate cAMP, we come to the conclusion that protein hormones do nothing more than stimulate the various

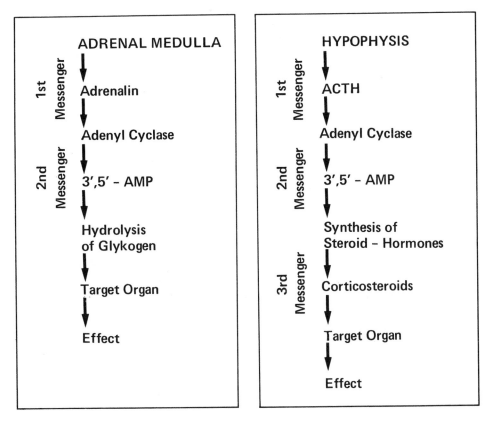

Fig. 4–3 and 4–4. Hormone systems with two and three messengers.

cells to perform the functions they were designed for in the first place. In other words, even the most complex protein hormone can only alter the level of cell-specific activity, but cannot change its nature. Any differences in the effects of the individual hormones are, consequently, not dependent on the structure of the hormone but on the nature of the cell on which it acts. This in turn, as we have seen, is a matter of the presence of a specific hormone receptor located on the outside of the cell wall, which picks out the appropriate hormone from among those in circulation.

In the final analysis, this means that a cell susceptible to protein hormone activation can never do anything, all its life, other than perform the work it was born to do. The hormone only influences its level of activity, but the cell can never—and this is the point—react differently to different situations, even if it should become responsive to several protein hormones, which is not the case.

Considering the protein hormones in light of this knowledge, we understand indeed that their basic activity (setting aside their stimulation of the steroids) is never situation-specific. The hormones of the thyroid gland and the pancreas, for instance, stimulate an already existing activity in the same manner as growth hormone or adrenaline; LH and FSH dispassionately stimulate the development of germ cells, be they ova or spermatozoa.

Looking at the steroids by comparison, we observe that the cells of the vagina and the uterus respond differently to progesterone and estrogen, just as the brain and the primordial sexual rudiments are capable of entirely different structural development, depending on the acting steroid. It appears that the steroid hormones are capable of stimulating *identical* cells to perform *different* tasks. This is their salient feature.

Having arrived at this conclusion through comparison with the protein hormones, we sense that this capability, to stimulate the same cell in different ways, must have something to do with the specific structure of the molecule. If we are then still wondering how the many thousands of steroids, with a thousand different effects, can look so similar, we must suspect that somehow there is more to this simple-looking molecule than we originally assumed. The solution to the steroid mystery, therefore, appears to center around the structure of the molecule.

The only branch of science that can help us examine this aspect is molecular biology. We must, therefore, take a moment to look into it, as far as it deals with the steroids. However, any reader harboring an aversion to chemistry should feel free to skip the next section without thinking twice about it.

HELP FROM MOLECULAR BIOLOGY

Molecules are like hands.

Chemistry frequently has to resort to terms such as redox potential, pH, dissociation constant, covalent bond, etc., to explain the mode of reaction of a molecule. None of this is necessary to understand the unique character of the steroid molecule. One need not understand the mechanics of a pin-tumbler lock to be able to grasp the principle of a key—and steroids are keys that are capable of opening certain locks.

Perhaps comparing them to hands serves as an even more appropriate analogy, for hands can perform very complex functions. As our hand consists of a palm that has fingers attached to it, so the steroid molecule consists of the steroidal skeleton with various functional groups attached. The hand's capability to perform a certain function depends on the way in which it is bent, and on the position of its fingers in space. Similarly, the functional characteristics of the steroid molecule are determined by the shape of its nucleus and the relative positions of its attachments in space.

This analogy may even be carried one step further: just as we have a right and a left hand, identical in every detail, there are steroids that are like object and mirror image. This represents a new way of perceiving the steroid molecule which, up to now, we have been visualizing as a flat disc. In fact, however, this disc is slightly puckered with methyl or hydroxyl groups, or single hydrogen atoms projecting either to the front or to the rear. Why? This has something to do with the tendency of an individual carbon atom to extend its four arms as evenly spaced as possible. If it succeeds, the angle formed between any pair of arms will be the tetrahedral angle, roughly 109°.

Whenever six carbon atoms form a ring, such as in cyclohexane, it makes sense that the two arms by which each atom holds on to two others must form angles of 120°, angles that are wider than the "comfortable" 109° (see Fig. 4–5). In five-membered rings, the situation is similar, although the angles between bonds are somewhat smaller. Such unnatural angles place the entire ring under a strain, known as Baeyer strain. In order to escape this angle strain, two carbon atoms at opposite ends of the ring flip up, while the remaining four move closer toward the center and, *voilà*, all the bond angles are once again a comfortable 109°. Now the molecule is no longer flat, but has turned-up ends. This shape is known as the boat conformation and, viewed in perspective, is shown in Fig. 4–6.

In the basic cyclohexane ring, those hydrogen atoms attached to the carbon atoms either project up and down, perpendicular to the molecular plane (axial bonds), or they extend outward, parallel to the molecular plane (equatorial bonds).

Now, as soon as the ring assumes the boat conformation, it is faced with a new problem: the axial hydrogen atoms which project in the same direction and carry identical electrical charges repel each other and consequently pull on the six-membered ring. This is called nonbonded interaction and eventually causes the ring to settle into the chair conformation (or, in the case of a five-membered ring, a conformation that resembles an open envelope), in which the hydrogen atoms are staggered and no longer interfere with each other

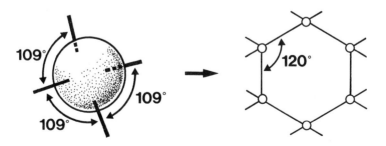

Fig. 4–5. Normal and strained carbon bonds.

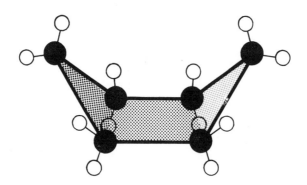

Fig. 4-6. Boat conformation (*black* = carbon atoms, *white* = hydrogen atoms).

(see Fig. 4–7). Since, at the same time, the carbon bond angles of 109° are maintained, this is the most stable conformation occurring in nature. All steroids that are essential to man, therefore, have the chair conformation in the individual rings that make up their skeletal ring system.

Since it makes a difference whether, for instance, a methyl group (CH_3-) projects from the ring toward the front or toward the rear, it became necessary to invent a designation for these two alternate positions. Those arms which project from the molecular plane toward the front (i.e., toward the observer), are called β-oriented; those which project toward the rear are α-oriented (as illustrated, for instance, in Fig. 4–13).

Double bonds, frequently present between C-5 and C-6, exert an additional influence on the eventual conformation. They restrict the ring's flexibility. One double bond means added rigidity on one side only, so that the resultant conformation is a so-called half-chair (see Fig. 4–8). Two double

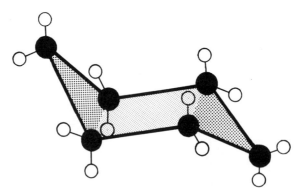

Fig. 4-7. Chair conformation

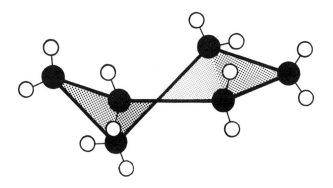

Fig. 4-8. Half-chair.

bonds (as for instance, in ring A of the estrogens) provide this ring with so much rigidity that it remains planar, opposing the Baeyer strain.

This insight into the architecture of the steroids meant a giant step toward understanding their mechanism of action. Today, any discussion between experts in this field would be unthinkable without an implicit awareness of steric conformation.

The described three-dimensional arrangements of six-membered rings had been proposed by Hermann Sachse around the turn of the century, but it took 60 years until they were confirmed by Barton and Hassel, who received the 1969 Nobel Prize for their work. Barton and Hassel applied the conformational concept of the individual six-carbon ring to the steroidal ring system, thus laying the foundation for the advances of the past few years.

Let us take a look to see how conformational considerations apply to the make-up of the steroid nucleus. It makes sense that in a cyclohexane ring, two of the carbon atom arms attached to hydrogen atoms, can just as well hold on to two carbon atoms of another ring instead. This is how multiple rings, as in the steroids, are formed. In this process, each individual ring retains its chair conformation.

There are two ways to accomplish this ring-to-ring fusion: either two equatorial arms hold on to each other, or an equatorial arm of one ring forms a bond with an axial arm of the other. Of the two pairs of carbon atoms that join in ring-to-ring fusion, one pair *invariably* forms an equatorial-equatorial bond. The difference resides in the second pair: if it, likewise, forms an equatorial-equatorial bond, the result is called *trans* (or *anti*) fusion (see Fig. 4-9). This is the architecture that is typical of cholesterol and the hormones derived from it.

However, there is an alternate possibility. If an equatorial and an axial arm hold on to each other, and if this happens between rings A and B, the result is shown in Fig. 4-10. This arrangement is called *cis* (or *syn*) fusion

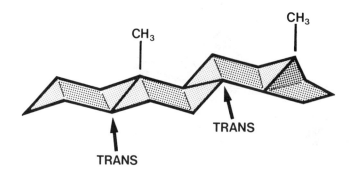

Fig. 4–9. 5α-Androstane.

and, as illustrated in Fig. 4–10, it changes the shape of the molecule considerably. As a matter of fact, these steroids suddenly produce entirely different effects. This is the nuclear ring system of the bile acids and the insect ecdysones.

An additional *cis* fusion, between the C and D rings, instantaneously produces an entirely different biological activity, this time directed toward the heart. It is the nuclear ring system of the cardiac-active glycosides and is shown in Fig. 4–11.

Experimental production of an additional *cis* fusion between rings B and C has also been attempted, for instance with progesterone and testosterone, in hopes of discovering potentially different physiological activities. The substances thus synthesized (not found in nature) were named retrosteroids (see Fig. 4–12). In some cases, these substances have been found to change an originally inhibitory effect on the hypophysis into a stimulatory one.

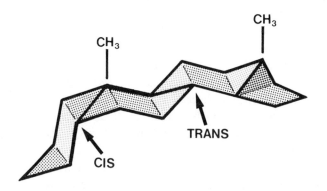

Fig. 4–10. 5β-Androstane (coprostane).

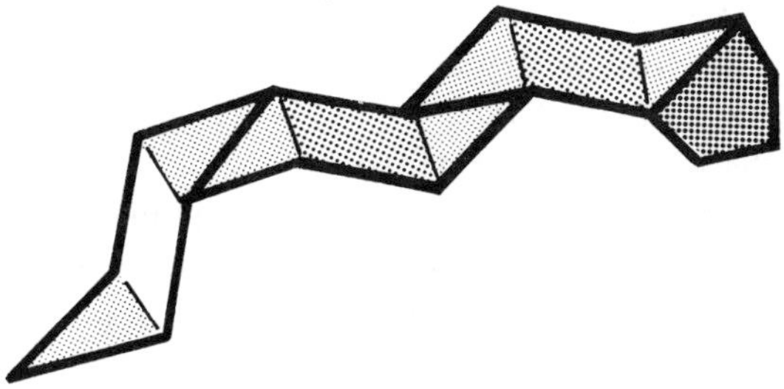

Fig. 4–11. Cardiac glycoside genin.

The above information boils down to the first amazing fact: without changing the "formula" of the steroid in the least, widely diverse physiological activities can be obtained merely by bending or twisting the skeletal ring system, i.e., the "hand," in different ways. The steroid molecule, which we initially visualized as a flat disc, begins to take shape: the individual rings turn into chairs, the whole molecule into a stairway or a rearing dragon!

The position of the "fingers," i.e., the configuration of functional groups, further refines the molecule's specificity. We have already learned that projection of carbon atom arms toward the front is described as β-oriented, while projection to the rear is called α-oriented. A substituent, replacing one of the hydrogen atoms that are attached to these arms, does not always have a choice of orientation. However, where it does, for example at C-3, C-16 or C-17, it makes a great difference, which one of the two possible orientations it chooses. For instance, a methyl group substituted at C-16 and projecting to the rear will mean high corticoid activity. If the same methyl group projects toward the front, the substance is inactive.

In conclusion, we need to say a few words about "right" and "left" hands. All naturally occurring steroids rotate the plane of polarized light to the right. It is possible, however, to manufacture steroids that are levorotatory.

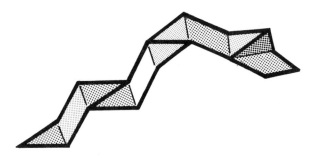

Fig. 4–12. Retrosteroid.

Analysis discloses that these are the exact mirror images (enantiomers) of the corresponding dextrorotatory steroids—just as the left hand is the mirror image of the right (see Fig. 4–13).

As already mentioned, these mirror-image substances are physiologically inactive. This makes sense when we compare them to the dextrorotatory types as far as steric architecture is concerned. An example of an *enantio-steroid* is shown in Fig. 4–14. It is obvious that such a molecule, encountering a receptor, has "all the curves on the wrong side," and will not be accepted. Welcoming a visitor, we will readily shake a small hand, a weak hand, or even a hand with only four fingers, but if someone offers his left hand, we are faced with a problem.

We should visualize a similar situation for the proteins that are supposed to interact with the steroids. They have clefts that accommodate the steroids and crevices that are a perfect fit for the attached atoms and groups. Far from being a mere didactic analogy, this description reflects actual bio-molecular research findings.

According to the most recent evidence, the steroid hormones apparently bind to the receptor with their alpha side (rear), while their beta side simultaneously wards off attacks. On their alpha side, their arms penetrate into the crevices of the receptor proteins, into which other molecules cannot fit. There, deep inside, they perform their actual chemical function which is determined by the nature of their functional groups.

We have mentioned these receptors before. They play an important role in the life of the steroids. The first meeting takes place when the steroids leave their site of production and begin to circulate in the blood. Specific "carrier" proteins serve the sole purpose of protecting the steroid on its long journey to "its" cell. Protection is indeed necessary, since there are not enough hormone molecules to allow for destruction of large numbers:

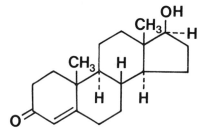 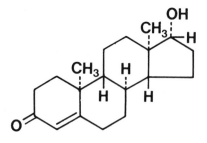

Fig. 4–13. Steroid and mirror image (enantiomer): *full-line bonds* = β-oriented, *dotted bonds* = α-oriented.

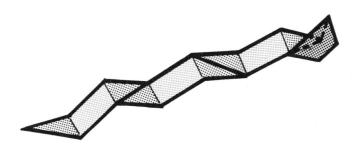

Fig. 4–14. *enantio*-5α-Androstane.

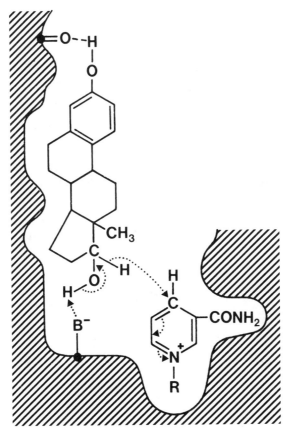

Fig. 4–15. Estrone, fitted into the cleft of an enzyme.

100 cm³ milliliters (ml) of blood contain no more than thirty-billionths of a gram of aldosterone. This means that there is one steroid molecule to roughly three billion other molecules.

Let us consider what happens, for example, to the normal daily dose of a standard estrogen (ethynylestradiol), as contained in several of "the pills" currently on the market. Part of this 20 microgram (μg) dose (twenty-millionths of a gram) is lost in the intestinal tract. The rest is distributed in 42 l of body fluids, attacked by enzymes, accumulated and hidden away in fat deposits, degraded by the liver, and excreted by the kidney. Under these circumstances, it is surprising that even a single molecule is left to reach the many millions of target cells in the vagina, the uterus or the mammary glands.

Nevertheless, it works. Of course, the carrier protein must release the steroid from protective custody as soon as the target organ is reached. The cells awaiting these hormones solve this problem elegantly by keeping available, in their membranes, another kind of protein which is a thousand times more attractive to the steroid than the carrier protein in the blood. The next step happens as quickly as though a pile of sand were searched for traces of iron by means of a magnet. It is as if the entire world population were herded through a mountain pass, and a specific individual could be picked out within a matter of minutes.

The fact that it is indeed the physical dimensions of the molecule that determine its effects, is nicely illustrated by stilbestrol. This is a synthetic molecule which has estrogenic activity and does in fact bind to the estrogen receptors of the cell. At first glance, it appears to have nothing in common with the steroids, but actually, the molecule arranges itself in a form where the distances between atoms correspond to those found in the steroids. In this form, it immediately reminds us of a steroid (see Figs. 4–16 and 4–17).

However, how do the steroids manage to penetrate the cell membrane

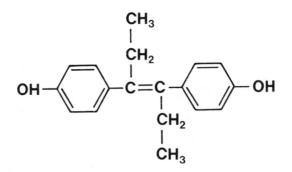

Fig. 4-16. Diethylstilbestrol (conventional drawing).

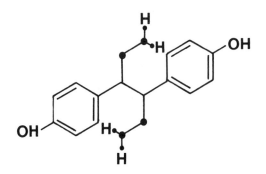

Fig. 4-17. Diethylstilbestrol (re-arranged).

which bars even the small adrenaline molecule? The answer probably has something to do with cholesterol which is a component of the cell membrane and more readily permits its steroid relatives to enter. It is assumed that the steroid molecule uses its "saw-blade edge," consisting of carbon atoms 1, 11, 12 and 17, to enter the cell by sliding through the cholesterol gap. This ability to slip through the membrane is a tremendously important property of the steroids. We have already learned how the fatty acids take advantage of this characteristic in diffusing through the intestinal wall, sandwiched between two bile acid molecules. Similarly, in the case of the cardiac glycosides, a sugar residue and a lactone residue have no difficulty entering the cardiac cell to induce an intensified contraction, as long as they are accompanied by a steroid molecule.

This permeability of the biological membrane to the steroids provides a first explanation of their advantages as compared to the protein hormones. Steroids have no need to send their message into the cell through the AMP mechanism. They can perform their task without the help of a mediator.

But what is this task? What is the steroid molecule, synthesized and protected with so much care, trying to accomplish inside the cell? We can sense that here lies the answer to our many questions. However, first we must go back in time, to learn about a discovery made in 1956.

THE SOLUTION TO THE MYSTERY

In retrospect, one might say that quite possibly the solution would still be eluding us, had it not been for a young man who, working at the Kaiser-Wilhelm Institute at Dahlem during World War II, happened to be interested in insect metamorphosis. We remember learning about this phenomenon in our school days: the brightly colored moth or butterfly lay eggs that hatch as ugly little caterpillars. During this larval stage, the caterpillar feeds voraciously and grows rapidly, while undergoing several molts. Then, some caterpillars begin to spin a thread a thousand yards long (we use the silk-worm's thread in the production of silk fabrics) to form a tight silk cocoon around themselves. Others rest in a hardened case, called a chrysalis, where, undisturbed, they are preparing for a marvelous event.

While this pupa, motionless and rolled into a leaf, or suspended from a twig, is externally quiescent, a miraculous transformation is taking place inside the pupal case—metamorphosis is without parallel in the animal kingdom. Then, one spring or summer day, the adult moth or butterfly emerges, enjoying the flowers and gently caressing breeze, and perhaps casting an incredulous glance at the fat, clumsy caterpillars, blissfully stuffing themselves with nectarless leaves.

That hormones had to be involved in these processes had been suspected for a long time. However, as we mentioned before: Who cares about an insect's love life or, for that matter, about its consequences? Well, Becker cared, and by 1941 his studies of the biological aspects of metamorphosis had reached the point where he was ready to let the chemists take over, to isolate the hormone and elucidate its constitution. In 1943, when he was drafted for military service, he assembled all his research results and handed them to Butenandt for continued investigation, before he left for the eastern theater. A short time later, he was killed in action.

Butenandt, barely 40 years old, with a series of successful discoveries of steroids to his credit, was willing to investigate a different type of hormone for a change. After all, prior to his discovery of the follicular hormone, he had already worked with vegetable poisons and thyroixine. He entrusted the work to Karlson, who had just completed his doctoral dissertation on steroids and was happy to be able to turn to something different.

The work took longer than originally anticipated. The end of the war meant relocation of Butenandt's group to Tübingen, but the project was not dropped. As a time when leadership in hormone research had long since been assumed by American scientists, Karlson and his predoctoral assistant began to process hundreds of pounds of silkworms in search of a substance of which no one knew for sure whether it existed or what it might look like.

"However," Karlson says, "the most urgent question was where to find the necessary silkworms during this time of total isolation from the rest of the world. It turned out to be a lucky coincidence that parachutes were no longer needed. The small German silkworm production became available. We immediately bought half their silkworms, separated the females (for recovery of the attractants) and, from the males, dissected out the heads and the tiny prothoracic glands for extracting."

Karlson reduced 500 kg of silkworms to several kilos of enriched extract

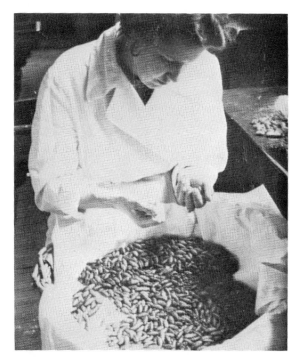

Fig. 4-18. The search for the silkworm's hormone.

which, in turn, yielded 25 mg of a substance he hoped was the desired hormone. The decisive assay was performed on March 19, 1954. It was positive: 1/100,000 of a milligram proved to capable of inducing pupation in the maggot of the blowfly *Calliphora!*

Chemical analysis brought a surprise: ecdysone, as the new hormone was named, did not contain nitrogen. We have already learned that, except for the steroids (and apart from a few tissue hormones), all hormones contain nitrogen. However, according to the preliminary analysis, ecdysone could not be a steroid; the evidence pointed in the direction of a long carbon chain. Looking at the physiological aspects, no one would have expected anything different. The process of metamorphosis from caterpillar to moth or butterfly certainly requires hormonal activities that are very different from those which the steroids exhibit in vertebrate animals. Besides, when the arthropods diverged from the other animals, very early in phylogenetic history, they left behind the capability of producing steroids. Insects cannot biosynthesize steroids.

Meanwhile, Butenandt and his associates moved to Munich, where they happened to meet Huber, a physicist and specialist in X-ray structural analysis. They examined, hesitated, examined again, corrected an error in the molecular weight, and suddenly all the pieces of the puzzle fell into place, spelling out, once again, the word STEROIDS.

Once more, the scientists relocated along with their project. After Berlin, Tübingen, and Munich, Karlson was called to Marburg. Hofmeister and the ecdysone problem followed. In spite of the small quantities available for analytical studies, the succeeded, in 1965, in establishing·the structure of ecdysone, which looked rather peculiar (see Fig. 4–19).

First of all, one notices the long side chain, which is similar to the one in the cholesterol molecule. In vertebrate hormones, this chain has been almost entirely degraded. Furthermore, the hydrogen atom at C-5 projects upward, i.e., the entire A ring must be bent down. This is a characteristic which, otherwise, is found only in the bile acids and the cardiac glycosides. And, to add the final touch to ecdysone's "old-fashioned" appearance, a hydroxyl group is linked to C-14, just like in the cardiac poisons.

Since none of the hormones of vertebrate animals exhibits even a single one of these characteristics, it is quite probable that the arthropods began their separate line of development at a point in evolutionary time when the decision to use steroids as hormones had not yet been reached. Once embarked on their dead-end course, the arthropods had no way of turning back. The sweeping and unifying wave of steroid simplification, which in the course of evolution ran through the vertebrate lines, had been unable to reach the arthropods.

However, otherwise, although a stranger to its own relatives in the vertebrates, ecdysone behaves like a true steroid hormone: it periodically influences the activities of certain cells and is, in turn, controlled by a protein hormone in the brain. In 1962, this brain hormone was isolated from 8300

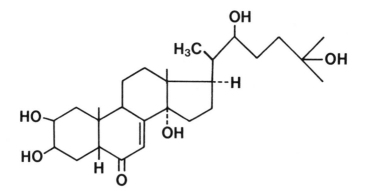

Fig. 4–19. Ecdysone.

insect brains by Kabayashi and his associates. Shortly before molting or pupation, the brain hormone stimulates a thoracic gland which, in turn produces the steroid needed to initiate pupation.

It has even been discovered how this same hormone can stimulate both molting and pupation, each at its appropriate time. In 1959, Williams discovered yet another insect hormone that he named juvenile hormone. Secreted together with ecdysone, it inhibits pupation and stimulates molting. Its formula (see Fig. 4–20), which was established later on, actually shows the carbon chain that had been anticipated for ecdysone. Was it simply a matter of chance that Butenandt's silkworm extract contained the *steroid,* while Williams had discovered the *carbon chain?*

During the course of this work, it was also possible to determine where the ecdysone comes from in these insects that are known to be incapable of steroid synthesis: many plants contain ready-made ecdysones (with slight variations) that offer themselves as convenient raw materials, or else insects can produce their ecdysone from other kinds of steroids ingested with their food. Because of this dependence on outside sources, ecdysone should actually be classified as a vitamin, but it has commonly been accepted as a hormone.

An overview of ecdysone's role in the arthropods (and that includes the crustaceans in which it regulates the molting process) is presented in Fig. 4–21. No one could have predicted that this insect hormone would eventually lead to the solution of the steroid mystery. It was just one of the many instances where pure basic research was to lead to highly important practical consequences.

To understand how it all came about, we must recall that, among the insects, we find a highly unusual characteristic, unique throughout the animal kingdom: giant chromosomes which are located in the cell nucleus and are the carriers of genetic information. They are much larger than normal chromosomes so that, under the microscope, it is actually possible to distinguish a succession of bands and stripes that correspond to particular genes. Probably the most-studied chromosomes of all are the giant chromosomes of

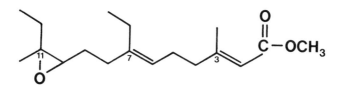

Fig. 4–20. Juvenile hormone.

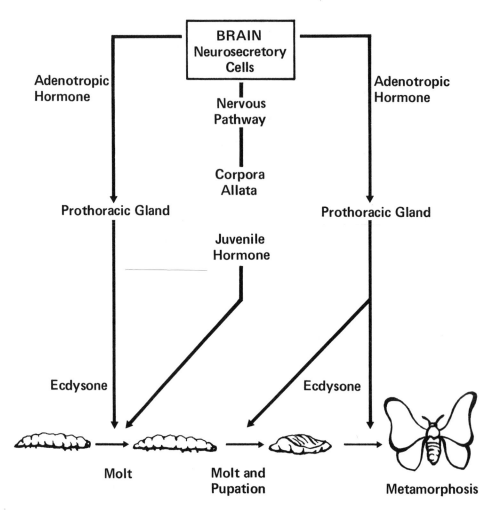

Fig. 4-21. Mechanism of the insect hormones.

the fruit fly *Drosophila,* in which one can identify distinct locations that control characteristics such as eye color or wing span.

Before we explain the association between the steroid hormone, ecdysone, and the chromosomes, we must briefly discuss the latter and their significance to the cell. In insects (as in man), the chromosomes bear the genes, which determine all the hereditary characteristics available to the organism during its lifetime. Its destiny is determined by their structure and by chance environmental influences.

The chromosomes in each individual cell contain all the information needed to assemble all the enzymes that will ever be required. Depending on the accessibility of this stored information and which of the many possible enzymes are produced, the cell will, for instance, store glucose or excrete potassium, end its life cycle or turn malignant in uncontrolled growth. Scientists had already proposed the general principle of such a mechanism a long time ago, but it took many years to determine exactly how it works.

What happened in the sixties, represents one of the outstanding accomplishments in the history of biological science: Crick and Watson discovered that the chromosomes are actually nothing more than bundles of long strands (called deoxyribonucleic acid or DNA) arranged in the now-famous double helix. Each of these strands consists of a chain of relatively simple substances, the nucleotides. They represent our genetic memory. These two young men won the Nobel Prize for this discovery.

It did not take very long before it was revealed just how DNA, which never leaves the cell nucleus, manages to direct construction of the various enzymes: it is simply a matter of a (negative) template, or transcript, produced from a certain segment of the DNA strand, which then migrates out of the cell nucleus to the ribosomes in the cytoplasm. This template strand is called RNA (ribonucleic acid), and because it provides a messenger service between the DNA and the ribosomes, it is more specifically identified as messenger RNA.

In the cytoplasm, messenger RNA attaches to the tiny ribosomes, the protein factories, of which there are many thousands in each cell. Small molecules, called transfer RNA, then select specific amino acids from the many floating in the cytoplasm, and deliver them to the ribosomes where they are linked in the exact sequence prescribed by the messenger RNA, to form a long chain, i.e., the desired enzyme. If the body needs a different enzyme, then a template is produced from a different DNA strand segment to provide instructions for the assembly of this particular enzyme (see Fig. 4–22).

One question, however, remained unanswered: How does the chromosome "know" which particular protein needs to be assembled at any given time? To explain this phenomenon, French Nobel Laureates Jacob and Monod came up with the hypothesis that a template or transcript can be produced only if the corresponding operator gene is active. This operator gene is located at the beginning of each of the many sets of instructions encoded in the DNA. However, since most of these instructions have to be kept on ice until they are needed, the operator gene is blocked by a repressor. Now, if the cell needs a certain template, first of all, it is necessary to bind the appropriate repressor in order to unblock the operator gene. This, in turn, permits

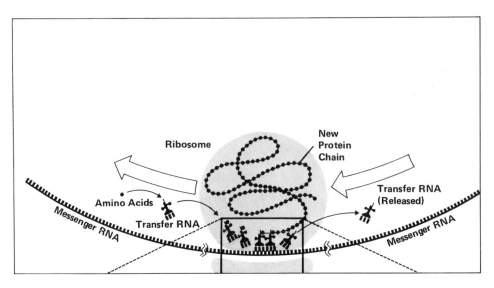

Fig. 4-22. Ribosome, utilizing amino acids to "knit" a protein chain according to the program provided by messenger RNA.

production of the template that eventually guides the assembly of the particular enzyme.

This leaves us with yet another big question: How can the operator gene be unblocked? It is true that some crude techniques, involving certain poisons or X-rays, were available for interfering with the structure of chromosomes, but these were roughly equivalent to the efforts of a caveman using a hand ax to operate a sophisticated computer. As long as the essential nature of the chromosomes and their mechanism of action were not fully understood, it was impossible to devise a method of influencing them in a controlled manner.

Then it happened that, in 1959, Karlson visited his former place of work in Tübingen. A geneticist, Clever, told him about peculiar "puffs" which he had regularly observed on the giant chromosomes of insects, just as they were preparing to undergo a molt or pupation. They both realized that these "puffs" were indicators of activity in the respective genetic locus. Since they apparently developed at the same time that ecdysone was active, Karlson asked, "Why don't you try and find out whether ecdysone administration will induce such puffs as well?"

Talking about this episode now, Karlson is self-possessed; he thinks back, calmly correcting a date. At the time, however, the implications that might arise from this experiment must have kept him in suspense for weeks. Finally, at Christmas time in 1959, he received word from Tübingen: 30 minutes

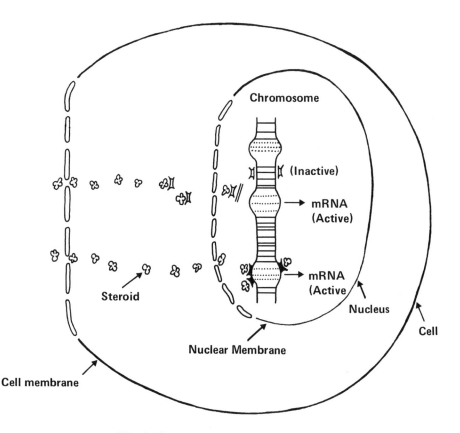

Fig. 4-23. Gene activation by steroids.

after administration of ecdysone, the chromosomes develop puffs—and always in the same locations where puffs had been observed prior to molting or pupation! That could mean only one thing: ecdysone had an effect on the chromosomes. For the first time, man had been successful in exerting a controlled influence on the genetic material.

Once this effect had been demonstrated for ecdysone, there was no holding back. All over the world, researchers immediately tested the known steroid hormones for this effect. Since the vertebrates are not endowed with giant chromosomes, this was not an easy endeavor. However, at this point, scientists knew exactly what they were looking for, and quickly developed alternate methods for measuring chromosomal activity. There was, for instance, the typical increase in messenger RNA after steroid administration; also, after transcription of chromosomal DNA had been deliberately blocked

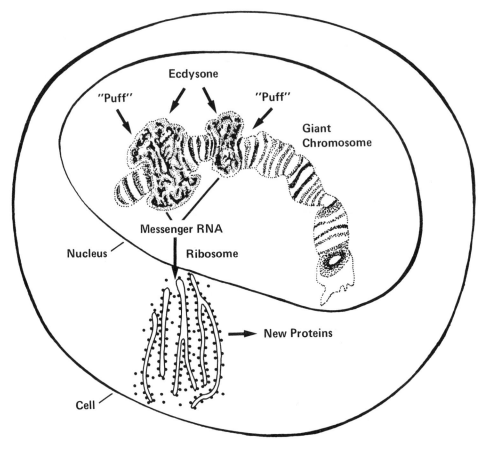

Fig. 4-24. Puffs induced by ecdysone.

(e.g., by means of actinomycin D), it was observed that steroid hormones were incapable of producing their usual effects. All results pointed in the same direction: the steroid hormones act largely by controlling the transcription of genetic information.

According to the current model for this mechanism, the steroid molecule (or possibly a chain of steroid molecules) either binds to the protective layer convering the DNA, thus permitting transcription of the corresponding segment of genes, or it simply blocks certain operator gene repressors. Perhaps these two proposed mechanisms actually represent the same process (see Fig. 4-25).

Finally, the reason for the steroids' fundamental role in nature had been revealed. Now it was obvious why the steroid molecule had remained un-

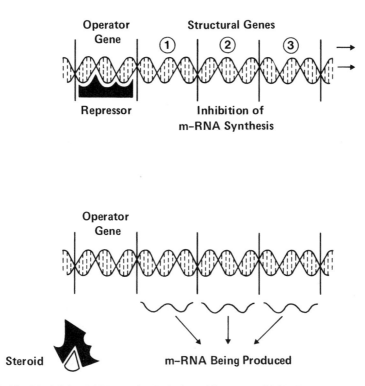

Fig. 4–25. Model for RNA synthesis, induced by a steroid binding to the repressor.

changed over millions of years of evolutionary progress: it had to interact with a substance that was even older than the steroids and just as unchanged — the genetic material. On that day in 1959, when the association between a steroid and the development of puffs on giant chromosomes was first demonstrated, 1.5 billion years of not-knowing had finally come to an end.

5. Houses on the Rocks

Deliberate Synthesis of Steroids

THE LONG TREK TO TOTAL SYNTHESIS

The comparison may seem somewhat surprising, but since the manifold effects of steroids may be compared to the spectrum of light, the steroid molecule itself may be perceived as the photon supplying the "energy" behind the many hormonal effects in our bodies. Thus, as the question about the origin of light has led to its artificial production, the question about the origin of steroid hormones has likewise led to their artificial manufacture, their synthesis.

Initially, science had left it to nature to produce the minute quantities of precious hormones needed for testing purposes. Progesterone, corticoids, estrogens and testosterone had been painstakingly extracted from ovaries, adrenal glands and bulls' testes or, in the most advantageous case, from urine. However, now that quantities measured in kilograms or even tons were needed, it was quite obviously impossible to count on this method for industrial-scale production. It had taken 15,000 l of urine to isolate 15 mg of androsterone, and the ovaries of 50,000 sows to recover 20 mg of progesterone. Synthesis was the only possible way.

In principle, there were three alternate ways of synthesis which even the layman can count off on his fingers: *degradation* of higher substances down to the hormone as such, *conversion* of very similar steroids, and *assembly* from suitable building blocks. In practice, all these methods were employed at one time or another, and in about the same order. This is easily stated in a matter of seconds, yet in reality, it took more than 20 years for synthesis to come to maturity. However, when the time did finally arrive, the ramifications were immeasurable.

These ramifications go far beyond the mere production of certain substances. Synthesis has led to one important development after another. Therapy is only *one* (albeit essential) reason for synthesis, so that we may end our dependence on the wasteful, exploitative extraction of organs and secretions. There are other reasons: synthesis confirms the assumed structure of a molecule beyond the shadow of a doubt. We have already realized just how important molecular structure is: it provides insight into how the hormone works in our bodies, how it binds to specific protein receptors (and only to them), and much more.

Moreover, the difficulties encountered in synthesis gave rise to the question of how the body was able to construct such a complicated tool, which had the best chemists of modern times baffled. The question about biosynthesis, in turn, made scientists wonder how this manufacturing process might eventually be influenced for therapeutic purposes.

The underlying reason for all this work, of course, is the application of "dry theory" to the human being. After all, medicine is nothing but applied research. Occasionally then, research opens up entirely new horizons, creating substances never before encountered in nature, where a minute change to the molecule may produce a totally new effect or permit the separation of naturally concurrent effects. None of this is feasible without the know-how of chemical synthesis.

Now, we all know that synthesis of chemical substances is a dry subject, calling for a very special kind of intelligence—at least that is how many of us feel about it. We forget that basically it is personality that decides on the outcome of an endeavor, much more so than intelligence. Intelligence is a dimension that we cannot identify with in another person, but we *can* appreciate the personality traits that bring victory. Neither the two Nobel Prize winners nor the mysterious man from the Tehuantepec Jungle, all of whom we will be discussing, would have exerted such a crucial influence on our world view, had their personalities been different.

It all started with Leopold Ruzicka, born in 1887 in Vukova, Croatia, son of an uneducated cooper. After his secondary school education, barely paid for by a provident insurance policy, he went through a period of intense soul-searching: should he enter the priesthood, or were his capabilities more in the direction of chemistry? Finally, he decided in favor of the natural sciences.

Many years later, he had a conversation with Pope John XXIII, who related that his own life had taken the opposite course—from the desire to become a chemist, to religion. There are other things these friends had in common: humble origins, the choice of a profession based on deliberation, the unconventional personality of the peasant, a certain physical resemblance, their eventual breakthrough to fame. However, it was much later that they were to discover their similarities.

At that time, prior to World War I, young Ruzicka set out from Croatia, went to Karlsruhe and, later, ended up permanently in Zurich. There, in a basement laboratory of the Swiss Federal Institute of Technology, he isolated musk perfumes—an activity that was initially more esthetic than world-shaking. There was no one to inspire him, no one to show him the way. He was always alone, working on projects of his own choosing, but he soon became an authority in his field.

One day, he came across the steroids. He believed that they were related to the perfumes he had been studying. Ruzicka was interested neither in isolation of steroids nor in their significance with respect to man; his specialty was devising methods of degrading or building up materials to obtain different substances.

"I had an improbable vision," says the lively 87-year-old, "that it would be possible, starting out with my specialty, the terpenes, which are constituents of many perfumes, to get to cholesterol and then, through dehydrogenation, to the hormones and bile acids. Natural modesty should have warned me against proclaiming such big ideas, since no one else had ever come up with the thought before. But thank goodness, humility was never one of my strong points; even at that time, I was stubborn. One day, when world-famous

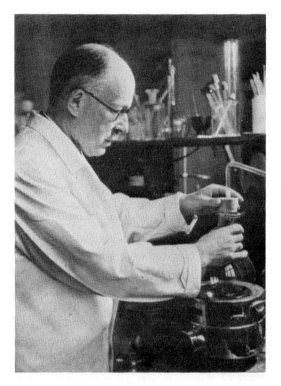

Fig. 5-1. Leopold Ruzicka.

professor Wieland was in Zurich, giving a paper on bile acids, I could not stand it any longer. A young man, relatively inexperienced in this field, I stood up and presented my conjectures without hesitation, although, at the time, it was not at all certain whether or not cholesterol and the bile acids had the same ring system. However, Wieland only shook his head and said, 'You are trying to accomplish *everything* by dehydrogenation. You are dehydrogenating too much.' I replied boldly, 'And you are not dehydrogenating enough!' "

Old man Ruzicka rises and, approaching his large window, looks out across the lake. After a while, he turns around: "But at the time, I did not dare publish my heretical thoughts. So the whole idea lay dormant until 1931, when Butenandt discovered his androsterone. While everyone was convinced that synthesis could be accomplished via lithocholic acid (a bile acid), I insisted on trying it my own way: via cholesterol.

"I was lucky. Ciba had provided me with ample funds (and thus also with the necessary assistants), and we had soon succeeded in synthesizing androsterone. We called the process "degradative synthesis" because it was accomplished by degradation of higher substances. We continued to experiment, and even produced some substances that had not previously been discovered anywhere. In 1935, in cooperation with Wettstein, we had synthesized an additional steroid whose presence in bulls' testes we suspected. A few days after publication, I received a telegram aboard the *Bremen,* informing me that Laqueur in Amsterdam had isolated the actual male sex hormone which he named testosterone. It turned out that this was indeed the same hormone we had synthesized—*before* it was discovered."

For Ruzicka, this was not the only high point. In his opinion, his subsequent synthesis of methyltestosterone was a greater accomplishment, intellectually, than androsterone synthesis, because it confirmed his prior theoretical considerations. For many years, it was the only androgen that could be taken orally without being destroyed in the stomach. "Besides, the royalties the company paid me, gave me a chance to express my gratitude to the city of Zurich that had naturalized me. I declared the royalties a gift to the city, to buy paintings and establish a museum. That certainly is a better place to display paintings than my home."

In 1939, he was awarded the Nobel Prize for his work revealing the relationship between the terpenes and the steroids. After the war, he continued to work in this field and, in 1964, his brilliant hypothesis led to the elucidation of cholesterol biosynthesis by Bloch and Lynen, for which they were awarded the Nobel Prize.

"And what is your opinion about the future of steroid research? Where is it headed, and what results do you anticipate?"

"The future?" Ruzicka asks sarcastically. "Do you take me for a fortune teller? No one knew in 1930 that steroids had a future; no one said, 'Go in this direction—do it that way!' People always imagine these things to be so simple. As though we had known where we were headed. . . ."

"To which quality of your strong personality do you ascribe your success? For you are a man of strong personality."

"That I always followed my own convictions without letting anyone interfere. In most cases where I was successful, I was *in opposition* to the accepted doctrine. I have such a strong personality, as you put it, that I once stayed out of the country for three years in order to avoid driving a nail into the coffin of a man in Zurich."

"And industry? It has recently been subject to increasing criticism for funding 'directed research projects,' i.e., projects that are in line with its purposes."

"Nonsense, without Schering, Ciba, Upjohn, Searle, research would not be where it is today."

He had never hesitated to speak his mind. We might have expected some controversial items from this valiant man's autobiography. Although he did not complete it, he left much that keeps his memory alive. To get a glimpse of his personality, we might take a look at the art collection he has given to the city of Zurich, and in whose selection he played a decisive role. Was it consciously that he preferred the baroque style of artistic expression, that somehow seems very compatible with his personality? He selected the most important Dutch and Flemish painters of the seventeenth century: Brouwer, Brueghel, Cleve, Hals, Hobbema, Rubens, Rembrandt.

Looking at these imposing figures, exuding strength and vitality, we recall the words of this great man of small physique, who said of himself, "I have never been a systematic person. I have always been an amateur with hobbies like gardening, painting, and occasionally . . . a little chemistry." He died at the end of 1976. Even *Time* magazine published a eulogy.

Besides Ruzicka, we must not forget to mention the many other scientists, particularly in Switzerland, Holland and Germany, who developed additional processes of synthesis. The list is too long to be included here. However, their work was of more than theoretical import. The concentration of steroid research in these three countries enabled European industry to be successful in the international market for the last time before the war brought down the curtain.

After these researchers had perfected processes for synthesizing steroid hormones, chiefly from bile acids and cholesterol, their patents permitted economical, large-scale production for therapeutic applications. In the United States, Parke-Davis offered but weak competition; Schering from Germany,

Organon from Holland and Ciba from Switzerland had soon erected strategic bridgeheads and, hence, controlled the manufacture and sale of synthetic sex hormones all over the world during the period preceding World War II.

This monopoly, combined with the fact that the price of progesterone was $100 per gram, obviously motivated American firms to seek ways of circumventing the European patents. Moreover, the German, Dutch and Swiss methods of synthesis, valuable as they were for the time being, were based on raw materials that were too costly for future mass production. Only industrial-scale production could have reduced the cost, but how were they to go about it? The methods employed for synthesizing a few kilograms in a laboratory setting are necessarily different from industrial processes which are designed for the manufacture of tonnage amounts. In addition, there was still the problem of limited availability of starting materials. The most commonly used method of producing progesterone, i.e., via cholesterol or pregnenolone recovered from urine, soon proved inadequate to satisfy rising demands. Therefore, it became imperative to locate raw materials which, on the one hand, were suitable for economical conversion (using newly designed processes) into the desired substances and, on the other hand, were available in abundance.

The obvious place to search was among the steroids that occurred naturally in large amounts, particularly among those that were as closely related as possible to the hormones. The first materials to be considered, in addition to cholesterol from lambs' wool, were stigmasterol recovered from soybeans, and the bile acids available from ox bile. They shared the common feature of a hydroxyl group located at C-3, which was needed for hormonal activity. However, they were neither inexhaustible nor suitable for high-yield conversion to precious progesterone. Consequently, the search for alternate sources of raw materials and new methods of synthesis continued.

The saga of the hunt for raw materials in the thirties has no parallel in any other chapter of the history of medicine: everyone joined the search. It started with Parke-Davis, recovering from their initial state of shock to prepare for a counterattack against the European patents. In this, they had help from Russell Marker.

The story of Russell Marker is the story of the "lone wolf" who was never paid what the world owes him—neither in cash nor in tribute. Without him, quite possibly, birth control as well as cortisone therapy would be accessible only to the wealthy of this earth. The poor would in fact have to "die young," as novels so aptly put it.

Because his story is so uncommonly human and because it is so enshrouded in mystery, one dares to ask him carefully, over dinner in Mexico: How could it happen that the many stories written about your life agree that you brought about the crucial change in steroid production, while, at the same time, the actual events are being distorted by the most fantastic rumors? Some reporters make you out to be the millionnaire consultant of large steroid trusts, others speak of your life in shabby hotel rooms. Some say you are dead, others claim you have disappeared. Obviously, all this is false information. Why is there this touch of mystery?

The nice, elderly gentleman with the hint of a goatee shakes his head, perplexed: "I can't explain it. . . . I only know that I did not contribute anything. Before tonight, there were only two occasions where I talked in some detail about events related to my work—once to the son of a friend, and once to a team of German newspaper and television reporters. Yet, year after year, the most bizarre stories are published about me, and everyone adds still more nonsense."

And then he tells his story, very calmly, very factually, starting on March 12, 1902 when he was born in Hagerstown, Maryland, a descendant of German immigrants. According to his father's wishes, he was to go into agriculture, but he insisted on his own preference and studied chemistry instead. Over weeks of laboratory experiments, he neglected the required paper work and, when he submitted a brilliant doctoral dissertation, was refused the advanced degree. Without much ado, Marker left the university that he had outgrown—without his Ph.D., without accepting the scholarship grant that was practically offered on a silver platter.

Within two years, at Ethyl Gasoline Corporation, he developed a method still valid today for determining the antiknock quality of gasoline according to "octane rating." By then he had learned just about everything that job could teach him.

In 1928, the Rockefeller Institute approached him with an offer to take charge of production of materials that they had been unable to synthesize. During his six years at the Institute, Marker published 32 papers on the relationship between molecular structure and optical rotation, a brilliant accomplishment at the time.

Then, in 1935, he encountered the high tide of steroid enthusiasm coming from Europe. Since he was more urgently needed for other work, there was a tendency to keep him from experimenting with these new substances. However, Marker finally saw before him something he had been seeking for a long time—a molecule of rather peculiar formation whose significance he recognized instantaneously. Now he had to choose: on the one hand, the safe harbor of the Rockefeller Institute, cradle of a number of Nobel Prize winners, where fame and prestige are almost guaranteed; on the other hand, the chance to follow his inclination. Again, he had no trouble making the choice. The Institute held its breath as the unprecedented occurred: Marker gave notice and accepted a minor position at Pennsylvania State College which, however, guaranteed freedom in his research.

At this moment, chance brought together Marker and Parke-Davis whose grant was supporting a research position at Pennsylvania State College. What awaited him there? A kilogram of cholesterol, no equipment and no assistants.

As a warm-up exercise, he converted the cholesterol into progesterone. In 1936, he used pregnanediol from urine as a raw material, employing a process developed by Butenandt. However, to Marker this was nothing but play. He fully realized that it would be impossible to increase production while utilizing urine extracts or costly, low-yield, cholesterol conversions. As far as he was concerned, there was no question that the raw materials for hormones had to come from plants whose steroids could be more easily converted than anything previously considered. Following an instinctual conviction, he clung obstinately to the sapogenins, particularly those found in the sarsaparilla plant.

What are sapogenins? Sapogenins are the steroid portion of the so-called saponins of which we need to know nothing except that (as their name indicates) they produce foam in water, so that they serve as the equivalent of soap for many primitive peoples. The sapogenins had never before been considered for hormone production since they have a long side chain at C-17 which is very difficult to remove.

Marker's first performance on the sapogenin stage was sensational: in 1939, he published his first paper on the subject, in which he claimed, in opposition to experts all over the world, that the prevailing opinion about the side chain was erroneous and that it was relatively easy to remove. A flurry of agitation and discussion of his work ensued. The resulting consensus was that it was "not worth mentioning."

However, by a simple and still common process (called "Marker degradation"), Marker proceeded to convert the sapogenin of the sarsaparilla plant into progesterone. To turn this into testosterone and estrone was child's play to him. However, the available amounts of sarsaparilla were not sufficient to support an industry.

Consequently, Marker bought himself a botany textbook. He learned that sarsaparilla is one of the Liliaceae, the lily family, which might include additional species containing the valuable sapogenin. There was, for instance bethroot which was an ingredient of "Lydia Pinkham's miracle tonic" against menstrual distress. Could this be a hormonal effect? Marker sat up and took notice. Indeed, he confirmed that this root contained an ideal sapogenin for progesterone synthesis, but again there was not enough raw material to warrant design of a large-scale manufacturing process.

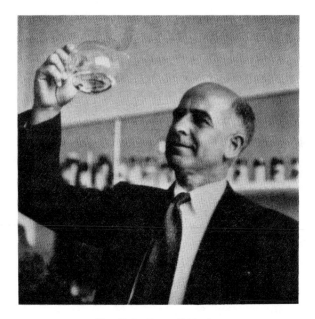

Fig. 5-2. Russell Marker.

God helps those who help themselves—the proverb aptly claims. Marker came across a publication from Japan, describing a sapogenin from a *Dioscorea* plant. It was called diosgenin and was, supposedly, unsuitable for conversion into progesterone, since the side chain was impossible to remove.

Marker immediately had a sample sent from Japan, established that it was identical with the bethroot, and, of course, succeeded in degrading the side chain, producing progesterone. However, how could one ensure a continuous supply of Japanese *Dioscorea?*

Back he want to the botany textbook: Liliaceae and Dioscoreaceae both are Liliales, a large order of monocotyledonous plants including, among others, South American yucca and yams. Over the following years, enlisting the aid of botanist friends, he collected 40,000 kg of various Liliales roots and examined their sepogenin content. However, it was Marker himself who discovered the most valuable source.

He had heard that, in Mexico, in the province of Veracruz, grew a variety of *Dioscorea* whose roots protrude from the ground like a bushy head of hair, and which is, therefore, called *cabeza de negro.* In 1941, Marker set out for Mexico, a standard letter of recommendation in his pocket: "To whom it may concern. . . ."

That he called on the President of the Republic was typical. He was referred to the U.S. embassy and gently eased out of the country. This happened a few days before Pearl Harbor, and rumors were floating around that the defeat of the United States would mean the return of California and Texas to Mexico. We can easily imagine that this was hardly the time to expect the Mexican people to put out the welcome mat for an American professor, intent on snooping around in the interior of their country.

However, with the naiveté of the scientist, Marker was back in Mexico in January, 1942. Since he had no permit to collect plants, he had to hire a native botanist. He describes the scene vividly: "First, the botanist came by himself to meet me by the small truck I had rented. After we had chatted for a while, he introduced me to his fiancée who was to come along. Then her chaperone; then her servant. What was I to do? I put up with this for two days, then I took off and drove back to Mexico City. From there, I traveled by bus, way into the interior of Veracruz. Finally, I found someone who actually sold me two large *cabeza de negro* roots."

While Marker relates these events, we are sitting in the famous Hotel Genève, where he was staying even then and where room 251 is always reserved for him. "I hauled my prize onto the bus, proud of myself for finally having realized my goal. The next morning, the two roots had disappeared! After drawn-out negotiations with the local sheriff, one of them was returned. Disinclined to wait around for the second one, I returned to Pennsylvania—the remaining root safely locked between my knees."

Marker found what he had been looking for: the root was full of steroids that could be converted into progesterone. This was the moment when Parke-Davis missed the boat. They declined to set up a small laboratory. Moreover, it was considered unnecessary to take out a Mexican patent for Marker's process. Possibly, it was fear of becoming involved in complicated patent litigations with the European cartel that drove the firm to this unfortunate move from which it was never to recover.

Angrily, Marker broke with Parke-Davis. He moved to Mexico to start out on his own: a loner, a stubborn individualist, a genius who was going to take on the world's mightiest steroid producer all by himself.

On top of everything, he did not have a penny to his name, although he had produced 3 kg of progesterone which he carried around with him. However, even in Mexico, none of the big firms wanted any part of him or his fantastic tales. Desperate, he studied the telephone book and finally found a name he was able to understand even with his superficial knowledge of Spanish—Laboratorios Hormona.

One has to hand it to the two owners of the insignificant Laboratorios Hormona. When a nondescript man plunked $160,000 worth of progesterone down on the table and asked, "Are you interested in a process for producing human hormones from plant sources?" they gave the correct answer. Together with Marker, they lost no time in incorporating a new firm called Syntex, one of the largest steroid manufacturers in the world today.

At the time, however, it was a one-man operation. Marker left the crude work to unskilled Mexican workers, while he personally performed the crucial degradation of the side chain. The first manufacturing facility for obtaining steroid hormones from plant sources went into operation in Mexico, using a process that Marker himself did not patent and which he would not allow Parke-Davis to patent later on.

However, for Marker, this state of peace was short-lived. He was an extremely sensitive man, unable to stomach the dog-eat-dog practices of the business world. In 1947, he sold his share of Syntex to the other owners for a song. Then he returned once more to the jungle, searching for new plants and new methods of steroid production.

After two years, he had learned everything there was to learn about *Dioscorea,* in the process discovering the famous barbasco root which had an even higher diosgenin content than the *cabeza de negro.* However, by that time, he had had it. One day in 1949, proceeding in his usual manner, he tore up all his papers, flushed $50,000 worth of steroids down the drain, and returned to his Pennsylvania State College. As suddenly as he had entered the field of steroids at the age of 33, he left it forever at age 47—true to his usual all-or-nothing style. "Since then, I have never worked in the field again, nor even read anything about it."

"What do you consider the proudest accomplishment of your life?" This 72-year-old man has an immediate reply: "That I have contributed, by not taking out any patents, to reducing the price of progesterone to one-hundredth of the original figure within a five-year span, thus placing it within reach of all patients."

"Many people cannot understand how you could turn your back on such a successful project. After all, it is you to whom Mexico owes its steroid industry."

"I have always done what I enjoyed doing. After I had solved the raw-materials problem of the steroids, the challenge was gone. There are other things that I find interesting. There is, for instance, the problem that many silver works of art of the French rococo period are preserved for us only in frail paintings or are kept in sterile museum environments where they remain inaccessible. Over the past few years, I have had a Mexican artist create copies of more than 80 such masterpieces by Thomas Germain and Paul de Lamerie—according to my own photographs. From this work, I derive the satisfaction of having saved something irreplaceable from being lost forever. That is just as important."

The quiet man smiles gently. "I feel that, this way, I have done something to benefit my fellow men, and it makes me happier than counting my stocks. There are so many things in this world that are on the verge of extinction, and I am trying to preserve some of them. For instance, in the barbasco areas of Chiapas and Yucatan, there are Maya Indians possessing unique ethnic characteristics. These tribes are now becoming intermingled with Indians migrating from the north. Similar changes are affecting the Zapotecs of Oaxaca and the Totonacs of Veracruz. A few more generations, and they will all have disappeared, with their high cheek bones, their broad faces, and almond-shaped eyes, as they have been looking down from the Mayan bas-reliefs for a thousand years. An outstanding Mexican artist accompanies me to the jungle and paints their distinctive faces to preserve them for posterity, while another artist simultaneously keeps the motifs of the Mayas alive in metal and multicolored enamel."

Silenced in the face of such fulfillment, we wonder if we would have the courage to get out of the rat race. An elderly professor from Pennsylvania State College did.

Nevertheless, life goes on, and individual personalities quickly fade into the background, particularly when they are quiet and modest. As far as Syntex was concerned, in 1946 they were simply faced with the question of what to do after the disappearance of the only man capable of removing the diosgenin side chain. Fortunately, at that time, a former student of Ruzicka was living in Cuba and, after initial problems arising from a confusion of names, was finally brought to Mexico. George Rosenkranz actually succeeded in reinventing the degradation of the side chain from the scant clues Marker had left behind. Within a few years, the one-man operation grew into an industrial enterprise that was capable of producing more progesterone and other sex hormones than the world needed. Only the corticoids resisted deliberate synthesis because there was no method available for maneuvering the necessary oxygen atom into the C-11 position. However, even the know-how for conversion into cortisone would not have changed the situation in terms of production—the amounts needed for treatment of patients with Addison's disease were simply not large enough to allow for a profitable manufacturing operation.

Then, in 1949, the picture changed dramatically when Hench discovered the usefulness of corticoids for rheumatoid arthritis therapy. The sudden demand for huge quantities of these hormones put enormous pressure on the entire pharmaceutical industry, albeit not quite unexpectedly. In order to understand this, it is necessary to go back a few years to 1942. In a last, desperate effort, tiny German interceptor fighters attacked American "flying fortresses" in the low-oxygen stratosphere. American military intelligence reported about "hormone injections" which supposedly enabled the German pilots to perform these feats. In addition, there were rumors about the shipment of adrenal glands from Argentina to Germany. It has been shown before, how in a special session of the Medical Research Council and the Committee of Medical Research, it was concluded that this could only mean one thing; the Germans were using corticoids. Actually, it seemed impossible. No one in the world could produce the huge quantities of corticoids required to inject every German pilot. No one? Well, there were Windaus, Butenandt and all the other German chemists. So, it could be true after all! As in the case of the "Manhattan Project" for the atomic bomb, a basic decision was made to institute a crash program. Review of the situation indicated that the Germans must have selected one of six active hormones. Which one?

It was decided to go for Kendall's compound A. However, even Thadäus Reichstein in Switzerland was unable to recover more than a few milligrams of this substance, and it required the adrenals of 40,000 head of cattle at that! In other words, what was needed was a method of synthesis: a method that could maneuver an oxygen atom into the C-11 position, since none of the known starting materials was endowed with oxygen in that position or close to it. However, there was desoxycholic acid which had an oxygen atom at C-12, and bile acids were available in abundance from packing houses.

Consequently, while World War II was raging outside, teams of scientists set to work in their laboratories, attempting to transport an oxygen atom from C-12 of a steroid molecule to C-11. Anyone unfamiliar with the related circumstances would not have believed that this was a project considered "crucial to the war effort." The goal was to produce 100 mg of compound A. Even now, we can identify with the research workers' motivational high, induced by the tripie combination of scientific achievement, patriotism and unlimited budget. (See also p. 87ff.)

Nevertheless, it took until February of 1944 to develop, in cooperation with Schering, a process that looked promising. Merck took charge of laboratory-scale production of the substance. Within 16 additional months,

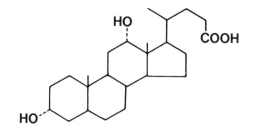

Fig. 5–3. Desoxycholic acid.

the task was accomplished: the requested 100 mg of Kendall's compound A had been produced. However, in the meantime, the war had been won, and no one was very interested any more. Yet there were still a few enthusiasts who were determined to continue.

Then came the second great disappointment. When the substance was subjected to bioassay, it turned out to be practically ineffective! It was only thanks to the stubbornness of three or four researchers that work continued despite this setback.

This time, they chose Kendall's compound E. By March of 1946, they had developed a process which required 30 individual synthesis steps. By this method, they processed 575 kg of bile acids to recover 938 mg of compound E, at a price equivalent to $12 million per kilogram. What could be done with this expensive hormone? If only there was a market for it. However, except for Addison's disease therapy, there was none—yet.

It was decided, *faute de mieux,* to hand it over to Dr. Philip Hench, who had already requested this substance in 1941 for treatment of his rheumatoid patients. We have seen how the results of this experiment made medical history.

The pharmaceutical industry, suddenly faced with a pressing demand, needed time to catch its breath. It was a gamble for high stakes, and Merck was the only firm willing to chance it. Even before the first successful tests were confirmed, Merck changed from costly laboratory synthesis to large-scale factory production and, in May of 1949, when the Mayo Clinic officially announced the miracle, they were able to offer the hormone, now named cortisone, at a reasonable price. Nevertheless, "reasonable" still meant $200,000 per kilogram. Yet, demand increased from day to day and it soon became possible to predict exactly the moment when the packing houses would be unable to supply the necessary amounts of bile. This was an unexpected development. Where it had previously been believed that price was the major stumbling block, it suddenly turned out to be the short supply of raw materials.

A frantic search for alternate sources of starting materials began. Demand soon hopelessly outstripped any amounts of cortisone extractable from available supplies of adrenal glands: Upjohn needed the adrenals of more than two million pigs to produce 50 g! That would scarcely have mattered, had a one-shot treatment been sufficient for the typical patient, but most rheumatoid sufferers were dependent on this medication for years on end, often for the rest of their lives.

At that point, a man by the name of Hechter had a brainstorm: Why not find out how the adrenal gland personally addresses this problem? He injected progesterone into the adrenal artery and was absolutely amazed when it emerged from the vein with an oxygen atom at C-11! What the world's best chemists could not do was accomplished with ease by enzymes.

For a while it seemed as though the problem might be solved by this method. Searle in Chicago had hundreds of fresh adrenals delivered daily from the packing houses, to circulate progesterone through them. The "steel cow" is what they called the complicated apparatus in which adrenal glands, freshly supplied each day, were hooked up to shiny chromium steel pumps and plastic hoses. This process provided a monthly yield of 50 kg of cortisone. Yet, with demand probably a thousand times greater, this was a mere drop in the bucket.

So it made sense to return once more to the search among natural substances in the hope of coming across some steroid with an oxygen atom at C-11. It was obvious that this could come only from plants. What followed reads like a detective story and initiated the greatest hunt for an unknown raw material ever seen in history.

It started with a reporter by the name of Laurence, who had heard Professor Louis Fieser mention that, somewhere, he had come across a steroid with an oxygen at position 11. Searching through magazines and old records of the Rockefeller Institute, Laurence eventually succeeded in connecting this remark with an almost empty sack labeled *Strophanthus hispidus* seed, which had been brought to the States from Africa 35 years earlier. Immediately, investigators pounced upon any and all available seeds of *Strophanthus hispidus,* but none contained any steroids of the required type.

After a while, it became obvious that although the sack did contain strophanthus seed, it was not of the *hispidus* variety. Someone, 35 years ago, had been a little careless with the label. After so many years, it was impossible to determine which of the many varieties of strophanthus had actually contained the precious steroid. So, the only thing left to do was continue to search, search, search.

Laurence was about to write an impassioned article, pointing out this important new raw-materials source in Africa, when he suddenly remembered that Africa was "under foreign control." What if these countries were to block export of the desired strophanthus seed, similar to what had happened with rubber and quinine? During an unpublicized meeting between the journalist Laurence, the president of the United States, and the chief of the Federal Security Administration, the necessity for a secret expedition was established. Additional impetus was provided by reports that Reichstein in Basel was also receiving shipments of strophanthus seed from Africa. (See p. 90.)

If we may give credence to the published accounts, typical cloak-and-dagger methods were employed to try and find where Reichstein was getting his strophanthus. Yet Reichstein, who had already helped the Americans during the war, was disarmingly naive and open; anyone was welcome to look around his laboratory, and take all the samples he wanted. This left investigators perplexed for a while, but then it was decided to outfit an expedition after all. Eventually, in Liberia, they discovered *Strophanthus sarmentosus* which did contain the precious steroid, named sarmentogenin. Since Liberia was "friendly" and there was no need to be concerned about export restrictions, the secret was finally revealed on August 16, 1949. The prize-winning article, which conveys much interesting incidental information (such as the fact that the cortisone yield of *one* ton of strophanthus seed equals that of 12,000 tons of cattle) tells of a "new elixir of life" that will help Africa and other underdeveloped countries. It suggests that plantations be established in Venezuela, the Philippines, India, and the Pacific Islands, where they would help the natives earn a living and, at the same time, make a real contribution to the economy of the United States.

However, this first government-sponsored expedition to West Africa had barely scratched the surface of the problem. As soon as it became known that there actually was a strophanthus variety whose seed contained the legendary steroid, industry was suddenly wide awake. As a result of Upjohn's negotiations with New York's largest plant dealer, the famous Penick expedition was sent on its way. Neither funds nor materials were spared while the expedition explored all of equatorial Africa. Thousands of miles were covered through Senegal, Angola, the Congo, Cameroon, Rhodesia, Gabon, Tanganyika.

This was the period after the war which we often remember with a trace of melancholy. The white man, fully aware of the superiority of jeep and automatic rifle, penetrated into the last unexplored nooks and crannies of this earth. With an air of good-natured condescension, he participated in the

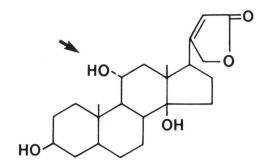

Fig. 5–4. Sarmentogenin.

tribal ceremonies of dark-skinned jungle peoples in order to extricate their well-kept secrets: the name of the vine whose pale, purple-throated blossoms fill the tropical night with their delicate fragrance and whose seed supplies the deadly arrow poison strophanthin.

In addition, a spirit of competition and secrecy prevailed, a hint of the Olympics and John le Carré. Merck had outfitted simultaneous expeditions focusing on Central and South America. From England, Belgium and France came the unsettling news that, there too, expeditions were being sent out.

In the end, all the romance notwithstanding, everything turned out differently than anticipated. When the various expeditions returned, heavily laden with arrow poisons, the situation at home had changed greatly. Meanwhile, in Mexico, after having discovered over 100 different steroids, Marker finally found one that did have an oxygen at C-12, which he named botogenin. In addition, he voiced the assumption that progesterone, available in abundance from *Dioscorea,* could probably be converted to cortisone. Since, moreover, more economical methods of producing cortisone from bile acids had been devised in the meantime, it was believed that it made sense to wait for perfection of a process based on progesterone.

To accomplish this in practice, however, was a different story. First of all, in spite of Marker's prediction, it turned out to be impossible to convert progesterone into cortisone. Among the chemical processes known at the time, there was none that could maneuver an oxygen atom into the C-11 position, as required for the corticoid biological effect. Position 17 or 21 presented no problem, but position 11 remained inaccessible.

Research workers at Upjohn started out from an entirely new premise. They felt that if there were enzymes in nature which produced cortisone or sarmentogenin with ease, then it should certainly be possible to find those *enzymes* in major quantities and induce them to transpose the oxygen to the C-11 position.

A strategic plan of action was drawn up, with several teams in competition: biologists working with adrenals, bacteriologists and botanists investigating enzymes, as well as chemists who continued to improve on the old-fashioned methods of synthesis. This all sounds rather confusing unless we bear in mind the underlying rationale that probably, somewhere in nature, there were additional enzymes capable of duplicating the process that took place when progesterone was circulated through the adrenal cortex.

The bacteriologists, headed by Peterson, won the race. As happens so often, it was chance that led to success. A culture dish containing a nutrient medium, left open on a window sill, appeared like an inviting habitat to a mold by the name of *Rhizopus arrhizus.* As it turned out, this mold was absolutely delighted to attach an oxygen atom to the C-11 position of a progesterone molecule. That was the breakthrough! A short time later, a bacterium managed to establish the double bond in ring A which is indispensable for estrogens.

This was the moment when Marker's economical progesterone synthesis attained its true significance and Syntex was able to test its capacity. Progesterone had suddenly become the most important substance in the steroid-producing industry.

Yet, the consumption of corticoids continued to rise month after month. It soon appeared questionable whether even the abundant supply of yam roots from Central and South America would be sufficient in the long run. Once again, Marker came to the rescue. In his travels through the Mexican jungle, he found yet another variety of *Dioscorea,* used by the Indian natives for fishing, and called barbasco. These Indians whipped the water with barbasco roots until the amount of sapogenin leached-out was sufficient to reduce the water's surface tension to the point where fish actually drowned, without being poisoned. This barbasco contained almost ten times the diosgenin found in *cabeza de negro* and took only three years, instead of 20, to mature.

This was important not only from the point of view of the patient, but also for the sake of establishing an international equilibrium in the pharmaceutical industry. The "small outfits" in Mexico were now in a position to offer progesterone at $480 instead of $3000, and had thus become the crucial factor in international big business.

Of course, this trend was supported by the Mexican government in order to ensure continued income from high export duties. In an attempt that is reminiscent of the Brazilian rubber monopoly or the Chinese silkworm, Mexico prohibited the export of raw materials in favor of expensive precursors or finished products.

However, even in Mexico, it is unwise to kill the goose that lays the golden egg. Pressured by this monopoly, the free enterprise system searched for a way out, especially since, in the fifties, demand kept growing steadily. Just as the European patent monopoly had been broken 20 years earlier, the Mexican raw-materials monopoly was defeated now: improved chemical techniques permitted utilization of steroids that had been unsuitable before. One of them is stigmasterol, another sitosterol, which is recovered in large quantities as a by-product of soybean oil production. The final, most damaging blow was dealt by the French company Roussel who succeeded in developing a process of total synthesis. Their share has already reached 20% of world production and will continue to increase, since the precious barbasco root—once plentiful, like our whales and fish—is gradually being exterminated.

Nevertheless, for many years to come, Mexican production will remain the most important factor. Yet it is true that no monument honors the man who was so instrumental in this development, nor has a street been named for him. All over the world, it seems, politicians and bureaucrats are too busy trying to immortalize their own names and those of their friends.

However, Marker harbors no hard feelings. He is back at Pennsylvania State College in Philadelphia where he first encountered steroids. Amused, but by no means resigned, he observes a world that would probably look very different without him.

The world production of steroids, measured in milligrams during the thirties, today totals 1500 tons annually. This is an almost inconceivable amount. To get a feeling for what it means, we must look at it in terms of the daily dose per patient which, on the average, does not exceed 15 mg. Let us work it out:

15 mg	=	1	daily dose
1.5 g	=	100	daily doses
1.5 kg	=	100,000	daily doses
1.5 tons	=	100 million	daily doses
1500 tons	=	100 billion	daily doses

Estimated Steroid Production
(tons of diosgenin)

Country	Source	1963	1968	1973
Mexico	Diosgenin	375	500	550
	Smilagenin	–	10	30
United States	Stigmasterol	60	150	180
	Total synthesis	–	30	100
Guatemala	Diosgenin	10	30	60
Puerto Rico	Diosgenin	–	20	60
France	Total synthesis	–	50	200
	Bile acids	20	50	50
Holland and Germany	Cholesterol and bile acids	5	10	20
Africa	Hecogenin	20	40	40
India	Diosgenin	10	30	50
China	Diosgenin	–	80	160
	Total	500	1000	1500

In all this, scientists did not forget that, in our world, there is yet another kind of synthesis which produces greater quantities of steroids than all the industrial plants put together. If we assume that daily steroid synthesis in the human body amounts to, conservatively speaking, 1 g (the amounts of cholesterol and bile acids alone probably exceed this figure), this adds up to 0.333 kg annually. With three billion human beings, this comes to 1 billion kg, or

1 million tons in man alone! This does not take into consideration the amounts produced by other organisms. The obvious question therefore is how nature, and particularly man, accomplishes this marvelous synthesis.

When, in the early thirties, the structure of cholesterol and other steroids had been revealed, the molecular architecture of these substances presented a tremendous challenge, as Konrad Bloch stated in his Nobel lecture. At first glance, it certainly seemed puzzling that the cell should be able to construct such a complex molecule, using the simple building blocks at its disposal.

It was therefore all the more amazing that, relatively early in the research effort, hypotheses were established which, later on, turned out to be surprisingly accurate. For instance, Ruzicka assumed at a very early stage, that there was a relationship between the steroids and the terpenes. Terpenes are substances that play a peculiar role in nature; among them are perfumes, plant hormones, camphor, india rubber and gutta-percha. Chemically, they are hydrocarbon chains which sometimes form rings. Their formulas are multiples of $C_5 H_8$ or, expressed in mathematical terms $(C_5 H_8)_n$.

In 1922, Ruzicka formulated a working hypothesis which stated that all terpenes arise from a common precursor, the isoprene unit. This is the so-called isoprene rule which was to prove extremely fruitful. The individual isoprene unit, a so-called *hemiterpene,* is shown in Fig. 5–5, on the extreme left.

Monoterpenes [consisting of two isoprene units = 2 × $(C_5 H_8)$], are found in more than 2000 plant species. In particular, they include the pleasantly fragrant essential oils of Mediterranean plant life. The two isoprene units may be arranged to form either a chain or a ring, with many possible variations (Fig. 5–5, center and right).

One and a half (= sesqui) of these monoterpenes make up the so-called *sesquiterpenes* [= 3 × $(C_5 H_8)$]. Here, the biological function is already higher than that of a simple perfume; for example, the previously mentioned juvenile hormone of the insects is numbered among these substances, as well as some hormones that regulate the dormant phase of various plants, which

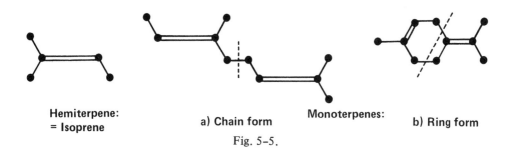

Hemiterpene:
= Isoprene

a) Chain form

Monoterpenes:

b) Ring form

Fig. 5–5.

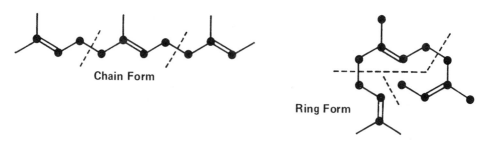

Chain Form

Ring Form

Fig. 5–6. Sesquiterpenes.

is accomplished by inhibition of DNA synthesis. Their basic structure is shown in Fig. 5–6.

Four isoprene units [= 4 × (C_5H_8)] join together to form *diterpenes,* including the plant hormone gibberellin, that also acts via DNA. The diterpenes can arrange themselves into various forms and if we take a close look, for instance, at the ring formation of tanshinone (Fig. 5–7), our immediate reaction will be one of recognition.

Finally, looking at the *triterpenes,* we will discover what this little excursion into terpene chemistry was all about. The chain 6 × (C_5H_8), called squalene, can form various kinds of ring structures, among others lanosterol (see Fig. 5–8). By dropping the three methyl groups at C-4 and C-14, we end up with the steroids ergosterol or cholesterol (see Fig. 5–9). In this group of cyclic triterpenes (also called tetracyclic, because they have four rings), we find most of the hormones of plants, fungi, insects and, of course, vertebrates.

Further polymerization leads to vitamin A, but still higher polyterpenes show less physiological control activity while the physical effects of viscosity and membrane hardening of the cells become salient. The gutta-percha molecule, for example, consists of 100 such units, while the india rubber molecule has 5000.

We are interested, in the present context, only in the assumed kinship between steroids and terpenes. If the natural terpenes arise from isoprene

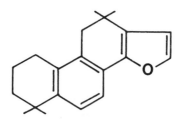

Fig. 5–7. Tanshinone.

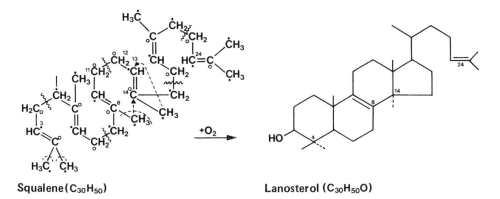

Squalene ($C_{30}H_{50}$)   Lanosterol ($C_{30}H_{50}O$)

Fig. 5-8.

units, perhaps the steroids do too. This fixed idea haunted chemists for
many years. However, assuming a relationship was one thing; proving it was
something else again. It is true that as early as 1926, there were some clues
pointing in this direction. For instance, there was Shannon's demonstration
that animals fed *open*-chain squalene responded with an increase in their
cyclic cholesterol. Consequently, it was assumed even then, that the mysterious ring formation might arise from folding of terpene chains.

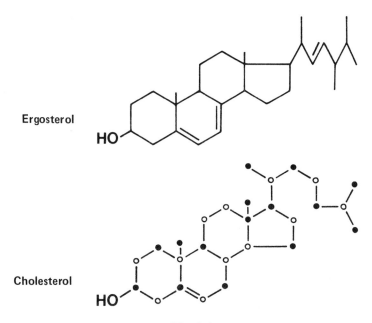

Ergosterol

Cholesterol

Fig. 5-9.

However, the assumption that steroids might be built up from squalene did not provide any clues as to how the organism was supposed to produce squalene. Even the origin of the hypothetical isoprene unit was entirely unknown. It was Wieland's school in Munich that had previously worked out the structure of the bile acids and now tested the hypothesis that acetic acid had to be at the bottom of this entire sequence. To prove this, Sonderhoff and Thomas fed yeast cells with acetic acid in which the normal hydrogen had been replaced by heavy hydrogen so that it would be traceable. Lo and behold, the heavy hydrogen appeared in the ergosterol produced by the yeast!

Unfortunately, the yield was rather small since yeast cells are capable of producing their own acetic acid, and utilized only traces of the amounts fed to them. As happens occasionally in basic research, scientists were side-tracked for a while, breeding new strains of various fungi. A certain variety of mold fungus finally exhibited the "deficiency" of being unable to synthesize its own acetic acid. When these were fed radioactive acetic acid, the entire ergosterol molecule turned out to be radioactive: there was no longer any doubt that it was built up from acetic acid.

However, it still remained a mystery exactly how this was incorporated into the steroid molecule. Then, in 1961, Folkers in the United States discovered a theoretically important intermediate product, mevalonic acid—the "missing link" of steroid synthesis, so to speak.

Immediately, a neck and neck race started between German-born Konrad Bloch in the United States and Feodor Lynen, in Munich. Even Lynen matter-of-fact and close-mouthed though he was, referred to it as a "contest"; at stake was the discovery of life's own process of steroid synthesis.

This race may have been more exciting than the outsider would expect. For instance, once, when Bloch was told that shark livers contain large amounts of squalene, he immediately traveled to the experimental biology station in Bermuda, where sharks were kept in captivity. However, this little escapade yielded nothing worth mentioning except, perhaps, a good sunburn.

Lynen also describes the work as "tremendously exciting," necessitating development of entirely new techniques for dealing with the minute energy changes that take place in the living organism. For this purpose, unknown enzymes had to be isolated in painstakingly detailed work—catalysts without whose presence the desired reactions could not occur.

While, in the United States, scientists demonstrated that squalene is converted to cholesterol, in Munich, the work focused on the steps leading up to squalene. The investigation was extremely difficult because the complicated conditions in the living organism precluded the use of acetic acid or squalene in their original form. Lynen discovered that a so-called activated acetic acid is required for synthesis of mevalonic acid and that this, in turn, leads to activated isoprene—a complicated pathway which, however, is associated with a minimum of energy consumption. From that point on, the organism proceeds in easy steps. In 1964, Bloch and Lynen were awarded the Nobel Prize for their elucidation of steroid biogenesis.

How simple it appears, when we read about it! Yet what a miracle nature worked at that time, in the Precambrian era, succeeding after 5, 50 or, perhaps, 500 million years in inventing steroid biosynthesis, and thus creating the only group of substances capable of inducing different activities in the same cell.

Bearing this in mind, perhaps the layman will not regret having traced, for a way, the footprints of Bloch, Lynen and the many others who contributed to our understanding of this important process.

IMPROVEMENT OF THE ACTIVE SPECTRUM

Separation into Component Colors

The original extracts of the adrenal cortex, the testicles, the ovaries, and even of the purple foxglove, had been *mixtures* of steroids which, accordingly, had a mixture of effects—sexual, metabolic and cardiac.

However, as Fraunhofer had separated light into its individual component colors, improved techniques of chemical isolation permitted the individual effects of the various steroids to become more clearly differentiated. This development gave rise to hopes that someday it might be possible to provide medicine with precisely aimed, specific therapies. It seems that such hopes have actually been realized in a number of areas.

Among the glycosides of the foxglove it was possible, at a relatively early stage, to distinguish between several substances, based on differences in resorption and excretion rates. This made it possible for the first time, after 2000 years of empirically based therapy, to tailor the effects to the needs of the individual patient. Similarly, by the 1940's, most of the glandular hormones had been isolated and, with few exceptions, assigned their fixed role associated with typical estrogenic, progestational, androgenic, mineralocorticoid or glucocorticoid manifestations.

However, the more one learned about these individual steroids, the more evident it became that even a prototype such as the glucocorticoid effect is a composite of many individual properties—incorporating the most diverse influences on protein, lipid and carbohydrate metabolism—which even include electrolyte-metabolic or sexual components to some extent. While it originally seemed appropriate to compare the range of activity of a steroid hormone to an individual color of the light spectrum, in time it became obvious that the hormone is a colored light whose wavelength is not quite pure—a light in which, although a certain amplitude is dominant, additional wavelengths are discernible.

Early therapeutic applications tended to look upon the dominant color as the main effect and the trace colors as side-effects. Yet, as doses were gradually increased, the initially undesired side-effects became more pronounced. In time, these side-effects, too, were utilized for therapeutic purposes, with the original effect then being considered undesirable. It has, therefore, become common practice to designate as side-effects any results that are undesirable in a certain type of therapy: the original principal effect of progesterone, namely prevention of spontaneous abortion, has been displaced by a side-effect—inhibitory influence on the hypophysis—which has now become indispensable for contraception. Here, in turn, the weight gain resulting from the original principal effect, the maintenance of pregnancy, has become undesirable.

Similar examples can be cited for all hormones. For instance follicular hormone, in addition to its feminizing effect, when used in high doses displaces testosterone in the cells and thus inhibits cancer of the prostate. Taking advantage of this activity turns the original principal effect into an undesirable side-effect for the male patient.

In view of such problems, we can readily understand that clinicians have been urging researchers to find or synthesize hormones whose typical properties, if not absolutely unadulterated, should nevertheless be noticeably dominant. In other words, an attempt was made to duplicate the achievements of physicists who had succeeded in devising sources of almost monochromatic light. The search for such "pure" colors by the steroid industry took many many years, and hundreds of millions of dollars were spent in the attempt to synthesize a purely anti-inflammatory or purely protein-anabolic hormone.

The goal of *one* effect for one molecule soon turned out to be more difficult to realize than originally anticipated. Research scientists did succeed in opening up the spectrum of the hormones to an ever increasing extent, and in synthesizing active substances whose main effects consisted of former side-effects. However, in large enough doses, almost all of the thousands of synthesized steroids still exhibited traces of unwanted characteristics.

Although a far cry from the neatly categorized separation of effects that clinicians had hoped for, this nevertheless represented a giant step forward. It had now become possible, in basically polyvalent hormones, to shift emphasis and simultaneously change the shape of the distribution curve. Any desired effect could now be respresented as the main effect of a molecule while, at the same time, the ratio between this desired effect and the remaining side-effects, could be optimized in comparison to the original hormones.

For instance, it is now possible to produce androgens in which the effect against female breast cancer or the stimulation of protein synthesis in bed-ridden patients is enhanced, while the masculinizing effects (such as those on the vocal cords) are minimized. Here, the location and shape of the original maximum have been changed. In place of a single, *broad* distribution curve, we now have two *narrow* curves whose maximum values fall within the range of the original side-effects (see Fig. 5–10).

It is possible to manufacture female sex hormones which preferentially inhibit secretion of the lactation-inducing hormone after childbirth, as well as others which, without any effect on the uterus, act only to inhibit the gonadotropins (e.g., in "the pill"). In the same way, among the corticoids that have been developed are those that attenuate hypophyseal ACTH in certain diseases of the adrenal cortex, as well as others that are largely anti-inflammatory.

Thus, steroid therapy has reached a degree of specificity that was beyond imagination in the thirties. Today, we can envision development of techniques by which it will be possible to custom-design a steroid's effects for a particular type of patient by manipulating the maximum of the effective spectrum in such a way that any unavoidable side-effects are simultaneously utilized to compensate for coexisting deficiencies. For instance, a convalescent male patient will be given a protein-anabolic steroid with androgenic effects and a female patient, a similar steroid with estrogenic effects, if they happen to be climacteric.

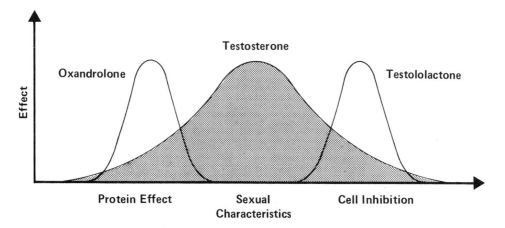

Fig. 5–10. Breakdown of hormone spectrum by means of synthetic steroids.

Amplification of the Effect

Next to specificity, what clinicians wanted most was a hormone that would be highly effective so that it could be administered in very *small* quantities. It has often been argued that it makes hardly any difference whether a patient takes 1 mg of a strong medication or 10 mg of a drug that is one-tenth as potent. However, this is true only to a limited extent. Increasing the dose of a standard-potency hormone frequently means not only an increase in side-effects, but also a greater amount of medication that has to be degraded by the liver. Although the liver is experienced in degrading steroids, a smaller absolute quantity to be processed will represent less of a burden. This explains why the clinician is partial to strong medications: he can use smaller amounts to achieve the same effects as with large amounts of a less potent drug.

The pharmaceutical industry has made great strides in accommodating clinicians in this respect, as will be illustrated by the following examples. Among the corticoids, the synthetic drug prednisone is about two or three times as potent as cortisol, and the latest additions to the glucocorticoid arsenal (e.g., dexamethasone and betamethasone) have 20 times the potency of cortisol.

Similar improvements were achieved in the case of "the pill": the potency of progestogens is measured by the so-called menses-delay test, i.e., by the amount of progestogen required daily to delay the onset of menstruation. Figure 5-12 shows how the progestational hormones have become increasingly more potent. The first pill developed by Pincus contained 300 mg of progesterone. By the time it was put on the market by Searle, it contained no more than 10 mg of a synthetic progestogen. Since *d*-norgestrel was synthesized, a mere 150 μg are sufficient to prevent pregnancy; this is 2000 times less than originally needed. Such figures illustrate the tremendous progress achieved in steroid chemistry, and the end of this search for the mini-dose is, as yet, nowhere in sight.

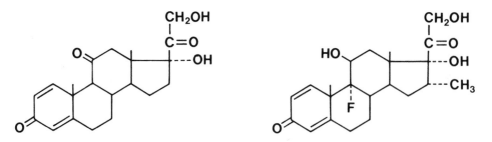

Fig. 5-11. Prednisone and dexamethasone.

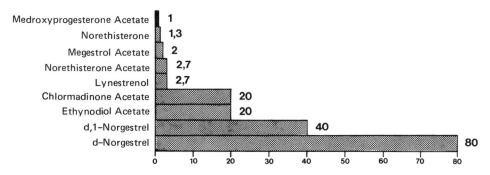

Fig. 5-12. Illustration of gestagen potencies of various progestogens, measured by Greenblatt's menses-delay test.

However, we are not always dealing with a "stronger" hormone. The superiority of the new synthetic compounds often simply results from the fact that, when taken orally, they are less susceptible than the natural hormones to destruction in the gastrointestinal tract. Or, because of interfering side chains, they may be more resistant to degradation by the liver or excretion through the kidney.

What really counts is the actual number of hormone molecules circulating in the *blood.* This number will be greater, for instance, when degradation is prevented, even if a smaller amount is actually ingested.

Whether the synthetic molecule's subsequent activity in the cell represents a true improvement in the sense of an intensified effect is subject to doubt. Like all hormones, it acts through the appropriate receptor, and it is unlikely that anything should be a more perfect match for this receptor than its *natural* steroid partner. After all, the two have been working together for a billion years and were actually made for each other.

If we return once more to our comparison with light, in describing these efforts toward intensified hormonal activity, we may say that after generation of the purest possible colors, scientists succeeded in developing high-intensity light sources with the lowest possible output of noxious heat, i.e., cold light sources.

Up to this point, the analogy between the light spectrum and the hormone spectrum is tenable. For a long time, however, it was an open question whether it would be possible to introduce substances comparable to light filters, which would reduce certain hormonal activities occurring in the body.

Introduction of Filters

If we look back to review the overall development since 1927, it is obvious that since the hormones were first isolated, all therapeutic applications have been based on two principles, both involving *addition* of the hormone: replacement of something that was available in insufficient amounts (e.g., in Addison's disease), or administration of above-normal doses (as in rheumatoid arthritis) to bring about effects that would have been impossible by means of the body's own production.

However, as much as 25 years later, the only solution in case of over-production, for instance of *aldosterone* in Conn's disease, was surgical removal of the guilty organ (in this case, the adrenal glands). Furthermore, what was to be done about sex offenders whose aberrant sexual drive was probably caused by excess testosterone production—other than castrate them?

Introduction of specific filters would also afford the possibility of suppressing the undesirable side-effects of hormone treatments, which corresponds to the blocking out of ineffective light rays in the infrared irradiation treatment of toothaches. However, initially, despite considerable motivation, none of the research efforts in this direction seemed to be getting anywhere.

A first indication that *suppression* of hormonal activity might be feasible occurred in 1953, when Landau observed that high plasma aldosterone levels had no adverse effects in pregnant women. Landau suspected that the aldosterone might be neutralized by increased levels of progesterone. Injection of progesterone into experimental animals subsequently proved that it was indeed possible to partially counteract the effects of aldosterone on electrolyte balance.

After the initial amazement had abated, an explanation was found rather quickly: the array of progesterone's effects includes a slight influence on mineral metabolism, which is present in much more pronounced form in aldosterone. This overlap of effects meant that the receptors of those cells whose sodium pumps responded to aldosterone, were also receptive to progesterone. Since progesterone has only slight activity in this direction, it is normally, for all practical purposes, inactive.

However, the situation changes drastically whenever, as for instance during pregnancy, there are sufficient amounts of progesterone in circulation to compete with the aldosterone. The two hormones begin to fight for the available receptor sites and, at a certain ratio, ineffective progesterone molecules begin to displace effective aldosterone molecules. Eventually, in spite of the occupation of all available receptors by steroids, the net effect on the sodium pump will be depressed. This mechanism, which is known in other areas of biochemistry as well, is called *competitive inhibition.* An interesting competitive method is employed, for example, in the control of insect populations: laboratory-bred male mosquitoes are sterilized by means of X-rays. When released, they compete for the females with the fertile males; although both the number of females and the number of fertile males remains unchanged, the number of fertilized eggs is reduced.

Accordingly, when progesterone is injected, it blocks the specific receptor proteins of the cells and thus makes them inaccessible to aldosterone. Unfortunately, progesterone did not turn out to be a suitable weapon against Conn's disease or other forms of hyperaldosteronism, since its slight aldosterone-inhibitory effect is overshadowed by its intense feminizing activity.

Consequently, researchers set to work to develop steroids which would be capable, like progesterone, of competing with aldosterone, but without exhibiting any additional hormonal side-effects. By 1959, they were successful: at Searle's laboratories in Chicago, Cella synthesized the spirolactones, and Kagawa confirmed their new function as hormone inhibitors.

Their most important representative is Aldactone (see Fig. 5–13). Today it is used in the therapy of all diseases such as cirrhosis of the liver, congestive heart failure and Conn's disease, which are associated with overproduction of aldosterone—resulting in excess sodium retention and dangerous potassium losses. Improvements observed in certain types of hypertension indicate that Aldactone might be capable of blocking additional, still unknown hormones.

Thus, the natural and then the synthetic hormones were followed by a third generation, the steroid blockers which are useful wherever the body produces an undesirable excess of steroids. The search for such "hormone filters" is presently a matter of high priority.

Additional blockers are already appearing on the therapeutic horizon. For example, scientists have discovered a *testosterone* antagonist, cyproterone acetate, which has shown promising results when administered to sex offenders.

Another steroid which is often available in the body in excessive amounts is cholesterol. Attempts have been made to prevent esterification of cholesterol in the intestine (and, hence, its resorption), by simultaneous adminis-

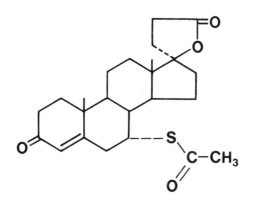

Fig. 5–13. Spironolactone (Aldactone).

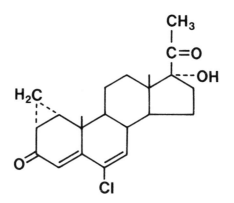

Fig. 5-14. Cyproterone.

tration of a steroid that is less readily absorbed, such as β-sitosterol, which competes for the receptor sites of the esterifying enzyme. Indeed, it has been demonstrated that a daily dose of 10 g of this substance lowers the blood cholesterol level.

In pigeon control projects, azacholesterol is used as a blocker. When the animals are fed corn impregnated with this steroid, it competes with incorporation of cholesterol into the egg yolk and interferes with reproduction.

Successful application of various antagonists has led to the utilization of this effective principle even in cases where a steroid excess, though suspected, has not necessarily been proved. This is the case for the gastric ulcers which develop as one of the side-effects of the corticoids. It is conceivable that "normal" ulcers, whose underlying cause is still being debated, might be due to hypersensitivity to one of the endogenous adrenocortical hormones. Although no such hypersensitivity has yet been demonstrated, there is a course of treatment for "ordinary" ulcers which involves use of a steroid. This may act via a competitive inhibition, heretofore unrecognized. The active component of the old-fashioned (and recently rediscovered) remedy, licorice juice, turned out to be a steroid. Its derivative, carbenoxolone, is one of the most effective drugs for gastric ulcers available today.

As far as high blood pressure is concerned, the situation is similar. Many scientists feel that certain adrenocortical hormones are responsible for hypertension. The remedial quality of Aldactone, which we mentioned, supports the hypothesis that this form of hypertensive therapy represents a competitive inhibition of unknown hormones.

Whether or not the effective mechanism in these and similar cases actually is that of competitive inhibition cannot yet be clarified with any certainty. It seems certain, however, that the future will bring the development of corresponding antagonists for each of the hormones. Such inhibitors will not only serve for neutralizing natural excess production, but will also filter out the undesirable side-effects of steroids used in therapy, in the same manner as optical filters do for light.

Even at this point, the analogy between the electromagnetic spectrum of light and the pharmacological spectrum of the steroids is not yet exhausted. In the process of seeing, for instance, there exists a dualism between the stimulating electromagnetic vibration and its physiological correlate, the perception of color. This gave rise to the question: What are the specific physical characteristics of light emissions that underly our perception of different colors?

Constitution and Effect

The analogous question was asked in the field of steroid chemistry: What is there in the architecture of a molecule that is responsible for achieving a certain effect?

This was a highly important question since there was reason to hope that the answer would lead to synthesis of custom-tailored steroids. Unfortunately, it turned out that there was no way of solving this problem quickly and completely. It has been possible, during the gradual unfolding of the active spectrum, to associate individual physiological activities of the steroids with distinct chemical properties of the molecule. However, attempts to use this knowledge as a basis for custom synthesis have not, as yet, been successful.

Nevertheless, some basic rules have been deduced. For example, to be active, the cardiac glycosides must have their C-17 lactone ring β-oriented (rather than α-oriented.) Also, a halogen (fluorine or chlorine) substituted in position C-6 or C-9 will provide exceptionally potent corticoids for treatment of skin diseases. We know, too, how to make a molecule water-soluble or how to intensify its anti-inflammatory activity (see color illustration on p. 13).

Some further rules are:

Δ^1—an additional double bond in the A ring—renders prednisolone four times as potent as hydrocortisone, at the same time reducing mineralocorticoid qualities;

6 α-methylation increases activity 2-4 times;

16α or 16β-methylation increases activity 2-3 times;

6α or 9α-fluorination increases activity 8-10 times;

16α-hydroxylation reduces activity slightly, with mineralocorticoid activity greatly reduced;

C-21 deoxygenation reduces the systemic effect.

Moreover, the following was also discovered:

Esterification with caproic acid prevents rapid elimination;

Breaking the B ring and adding a double bond between C-7 and C-8 produces an effect on calcium metabolism.

An oxygen atom at C-20 produces a progestational effect, while an additional oxygen at C-21 (and possibly C-11) results in corticoid activity.

An oxygen atom at C-17 influences carbohydrate metabolism whereas, at C-18, it intensifies the mineralocorticoid effect.

Degradation of steroids to 19 carbon atoms results in androgenic activity, while degradation to 18 carbon atoms leads to estrogenic activity.

However, apart from this, our knowledge is still very limited. Daily, we receive additional information about new synthetic substances that deviate from these rules or add new ones, such as the unexpected increase in potency through halogenation at C-6 or C-9, which does not occur naturally. Thus, there is no choice but to screen each individual new substance for any and all possible hormonal effects, a time-consuming process requiring the patience of a saint.

Progress was no less difficult in the final area of analogy between the spectrum of the steroids and the spectrum of light: after the wavelengths of electromagnetic radiation had been correlated with the perception of various colors, it was noted that beyond red and violet, there were wavelengths that apparently elicited no response in the eye. The infrared and ultraviolet ranges were optically "empty." However, it did not take long to recognize that the same kind of radiation that elicited color perception in the eye also had considerable effects on the rest of the body, effects that had not previously been thought of as related to light.

Very soon, one realized the relationship between infrared radiation and the sensation of warmth on the skin, as experienced close to a red-hot stove, and between ultraviolet radiation and tanning of the skin in alpine mountain regions. It took a little longer to recognize the biological effects of higher-frequency radiation: the therapeutic effect of ultra-short waves now used in diathermy to warm the deeper tissues of the body, the mutational effect of cosmic radiation, and cell destruction by X-rays.

If the hormone scientists could learn anything from this analogy, it was the fact that searching for new kinds of radiation, i.e., new steroids, was not enough. Rather, it was necessary to widen their horizon to accommodate entirely new areas—areas which had perhaps not yet been identified as hormonal, but which did respond to steroids. This meant, of course, that a vast field opened up in which, at times, one seemed unable to make any progress.

Nevertheless, it eventually became possible to look beyond the ends of the spectrum.

The Ends of the Spectrum

To begin with, we are faced with the task of finding the unknown causal agent of activities as yet unidentified.

Why is it so difficult to discover hormones that are still unknown? To answer this question, we must point out the almost insurmountable technical difficulties such a search faces today.

First of all, there is the choice of body substance from which the unknown hormone is to be isolated. In other words: Where should one begin searching? The solution that comes to mind initially is to look in those organs that are known to produce hormones and should, therefore, contain them in relatively high concentrations. This is similar to the manner in which the adrenal cortex and the gonads were investigated years ago. However, all the likely organs have been so thoroughly explored by now that unknown steroids will probably be found only in unexpected locations, such as the recently discovered vitamin D hormone in the kidney. However, to search blindly, without any clues, in *all* organs would be a hopeless endeavor. Keep in mind the difficulties encountered in the isolation of the corticoids, even though the adrenal cortex had actually been "suspect." Imagine, then, what a chore it would have been to try to isolate those few milligrams of a steroid from the total mass of 40,000 head of cattle instead of directly from the concentrate of the appropriate hormone "factories."

As an alternate starting point, one might consider body fluids for isolation of unknown hormones. We might begin with urine from which, as we recall, the first hormones had been isolated. Moreover, urine, which contains few incidental molecules, is easily extracted. Alas, it has been demonstrated that the successful discovery of the sex hormones in urine was a unique stroke of good luck. Many steroids have undergone metabolic changes by the time they pass through the kidney tubules; others appear in urine in minute amounts, or only rarely. Moreover, urine has been thoroughly investigated and seems to offer no reason to expect any startling discoveries.

Therefore, in the absence of a "suspect" organ, all that remains is the blood which is the vehicle of transportation of all hormones wishing to reach their targets. However, to search in the blood is a tremendous task, especially since any steroids that have eluded detection are probably present in concentrations far below that of aldosterone (which circulates in the blood in a dilution of one part to three billion).

The next question then is: What methods shall we use? Ever since the search for the steroid hormones began, *methodology* has always been the limiting factor. In the beginning, chemical processes, mostly color reactions, had been used for quantitative determination of hormones, but even that had been possible only in case of high concentrations. Later on, fluorometric techniques were developed by means of which, for instance, it was possible to determine the presence of cortisol.

The invention of gas chromatography permitted quantitative analysis of additional hormones, present in lower concentrations. Yet even this method was, initially, not sensitive enough in all cases: the famous Geigy tables of 1969 still contain the note, "Determination of estradiol in the blood is not possible."

In the meantime, however, it has become feasible to analyze steroid concentrations in the blood from androsterone all the way down to aldosterone. For instance, 100 ml of plasma contain the following approximate hormone amounts, with 1 nanogram (ng) equal to one billionth of a gram:

Androsterone	30,000 ng	Progesterone	200 ng
Cortisol	10,000 ng	Estradiol	125 ng
Corticosterone	1,000 ng	Aldosterone	30 ng
Testosterone	700 ng		

To represent this enormous range in a graph, we would have to use a logarithmic scale.

Nevertheless, since it was possible to bridge the thousandfold span between androsterone and aldosterone, it is not inconceivable that someday we will be able to find hormones whose concentration is, in turn, 1000 times lower than that of aldosterone. Even now, the method of radioimmunoassay permits detection of fractions of a picogram (1 pg = one-trillionth of a gram).

Is there really a chance of discovering a new hormone today, more than 50 years after the discovery of estradiol? It is not as improbable as it may sound. As a matter of fact, new hormones are still being discovered—more slowly, to be sure—but there certainly seems no end in sight despite all the methodological problems.

There are, for instance, the new findings about vitamin D which we mentioned earlier and which indicate that what we are dealing with here, is not the end product, but only an intermediary link, in the pathway leading to the actual hormone "1,25-DHCC."

Another case in point is the male sex hormone. At first, one could isolate only androsterone. Later, testosterone, 40 times less concentrated, was believed to be the actual hormone. Recently, by continuing to trace its pathway in the body, it was found that testosterone is not the male hormone in its final form. The active form has no double bond between C-4 and C-5, but two hydrogen atoms at these positions instead. This new substance, called DHT (dihydrotestosterone), is much more potent than testosterone and is synthesized in the testicular tissues.

Consequently, here we have two new hormones, possessing undreamed-of potency, whose presence was quite unknown even a few years ago. This gives us the courage to continue searching. But for what? Our body is full of substances in picogram amounts, many of them possibly quite uninteresting. How should we know which ones do or do not have biological effects? Well, to determine this, we must start out with some suspicion that certain physiological processes may be due to steroid hormones—as had been the case with the sex hormones. The search, however, is becoming increasingly more difficult, since all the obvious associations between diseases and steroids have been investigated. Yet even though the search has become more difficult, it is by no means over. There is much evidence suggesting that there are, in our bodies, certain locks to which we have as yet been unable to discover the natural steroid keys.

One such lock is the phenomenon of *sleep,* which is periodically locked and unlocked by a key yet unknown to us. There are many clues pointing to an unknown steroid, possibly a degradation product of known hormones. Such an assumption would be mere speculation, were it not for unambiguous evidence of the activity of steroids in the brain. We will recall how the water beetle protects itself against hostile fish by means of the steroid cortexolone which puts them to sleep. In addition, we will remember how the development of personality is influenced by the sex hormones, both in the fetal period and during puberty. There is, moreover, Addison's excellent description of the nervousness, insomnia and peculiar hypersensitivity of the olfactory nerves in disorders of the adrenal glands, as well as a certain euphoria observed in many patients who must take corticoids.

There are other clues which point to a hormonal mediation of sleep: to begin with, we have the curve of adrenocortical activity (measured by its glucocorticoid output), as shown in Fig. 5–15. Quite obviously, it is synchronized with the rhythm of sleep. It is conceivable that as the blood hormone level drops, degradation products, so-called catabolites, are formed which induce sleep; or perhaps a sleep hormone of the adrenal cortex is released a few hours ahead of the production of other steroids, to induce the necessary state of sleep.

Moreover, there are direct connections between steroids and sleep: in 1940, Selye injected various steroids into the peritoneal cavities of laboratory rats and found, to his amazement, that the animals went into a deep and apparently normal state of sleep. This required 100 mg of estrone, but only 25 mg of androsterone or 10 mg of progesterone. During the course of these experiments, Selye developed additional steroids, for instance 5β=pregnane-

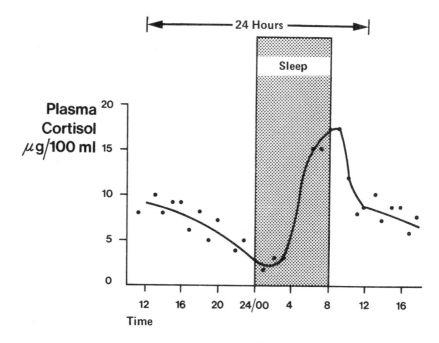

Fig. 5-15. Circadian rhythm of human corticoid production.

3,20-dione, which are 5-10 times more potent than progesterone. Is it not conceivable that the body uses hormones to induce not only the state of hibernation in the bear, but our own nightly sleep as well? So far, more than 100 different steroids have been identified in the human brain, their structures and functions not established in all cases. Possibly, one of them will turn out to be a sleep hormone.

Sleep is not the only lock that is missing a key. *Temperature regulation* is another physiological function which can be influenced by steroids, although no specific hormone has, as yet, been discovered. As early as 1868, Wunderlich reported the surprising observation that, in addition to its cardiac activity, digitalis also reduces fever in patients suffering from enteritis (see Fig. 5-16). This effect, forgotten for many years, has recently gained renewed significance in connection with measurement of the so-called basal temperature in women: along with progesterone secretion, during the second phase of the menstrual cycle, all women experience a slight temperature increase whose discovery, as an indicator of ovulation, represented a milestone in the early history of contraception, since it afforded a distinction between fertile and infertile periods (see Fig. 5-17). Here, the effect is the opposite of what happens with digitalis: instead of a temperature reduction,

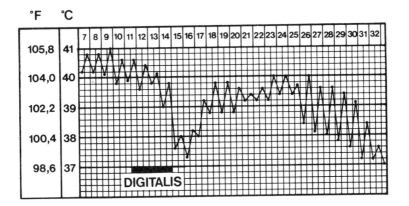

Fig. 5-16. Reduction of fever in enteritis after administration of digitalis.

there is a temperature increase. However, antagonistic effects of two steroids are readily explained by the process of competitive inhibition.

The increase in basal temperature is probably not due, simply, to stimulation of the temperature control center, as for instance in the case of bacterial toxins. This is illustrated by etiocholanolone, a degradation product of cholesterol and many other steroids: 12 hours after ingestion (after it has long since been eliminated from the body), this substance induces a fever up to 104°F. In other words, this steroid initiates a drawn-out process which eventually results in a rise in temperature. Such a delayed-action process is usually based on protein synthesis, which often requires several hours before the effect becomes evident. It is frequently encountered among the steroids and makes good sense within the general framework of steroid mechanisms. It is therefore not implausible that the periodic regulation of normal body temperature, including the lowered temperature of certain animals during hibernation, may be mediated by steroids that remain to be identified.

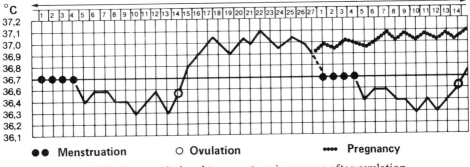

Fig. 5-17. Increase in basal temperature in women after ovulation.

Blood pressure, recently a focus of renewed interest, is yet another area in which control by steroids is suspected. It had been known for many years that certain hormones, such as corticosterone or aldosterone, can lead to an increase in blood pressure. However, while a few forms of hypertension can be traced to excess production of these hormones, it has been impossible to prove such a causality in the great majority of ordinary hypertensive patients. Nevertheless, several scientists investigated the possible existence of a specific blood pressure hormone, beyond the control of higher centers, which might be causing the "normal" hypertensive disease. Initially, there was very little evidence to support such a hypothesis.

Then, surprisingly, a clue came from investigations of the protein hormones that stimulate steroid secretion. The superordinate hormone for aldosterone, renin, is synthesized in the kidney. As already mentioned, renin has a feedback regulatory mechanism of its own: as soon as the blood level of aldosterone exceeds a certain limit, renin synthesis is automatically cut back. Consequently, in Conn's disease (where an adrenal tumor continuously produces large quantities of aldosterone), the production of renin drops to a barely measurable level.

As biochemical techniques became increasingly more refined, it was possible to detect that in a large percentage of "normal" hypertensive patients, renin production is suppressed long before the critical plasma aldosterone level has been reached. The obvious conclusion was that an additional, still-unknown steroid caused the renin-inhibiting feedback signal—a hormone that, at the same time, was responsible for the increase in blood pressure. The search for such a hormone is presently in full swing: 18-hydroxy-desoxycorticosterone is one of the steroids that are suspected of contributing to hypertension.

Consequent therapeutic success served to confirm the suspicion that this increase in blood pressure may be caused by a steroid: administration of the previously mentioned steroid blocker spironolactone actually normalizes the blood pressure in hypertensive patients with low renin levels.

Cardiac activity represents an additional, extensive field in which steroids may be physiologically active, specifically in regard to the force of contraction. This effect is called *inotropic* (in contrast to influences on frequency, the P-R interval, etc.) and there is no doubt that it is increased by steroids of the digitalis group.

The fact that "by coincidence" thousands of plants and even some primitive animals contain a steroid which is an exact fit for the receptors in the human heart muscle, inducing such positive and specific effects, is striking. We find it difficult to ward off the suspicion that such a "cardiac hormone" actually exists and that it should resemble digitalis as far as molecular architecture is concerned.

We will not go into the complex reasons that support the idea of steroid influences in other areas such as aging or arteriosclerosis. Nevertheless, it is assumed that the search for unknown hormones will, in the future, include these fields as well.

Of course, there is always the chance that some of the steroid hormones that have been eluding detection simply no longer exist in the human body, because man has lost the ability to synthesize them. This may apply particularly to the digitalis-type steroids which, phylogenetically, are probably older than our hormones. We recall vitamin D which we are able to produce only partially, while its synthesis is no problem for plankton, or the insects' ecdysones which they cannot produce for themselves. In all of these cases, the capability of steroid synthesis has been lost, but the receptors which respond to these hormones still exist.

Of course, we can carry this speculation even further: we may reasonably expect to find additional endogenous steroids that might be used for deliberate therapeutic intervention in vital physiological processes. Beyond this, it may be possible to design steroids to fit certain locks for which the keys have been lost, which, for instance, may apply in the case of the catatoxic steroids.

Once a *suspicion* has been aroused, linking certain biological processes with unknown steroids, the next task will be the development of appropriate tests. This will become increasingly more difficult as we penetrate further into the momentous field of chronic diseases—aging, arteriosclerosis, multiple sclerosis, hypertension. This is especially true since the steroids yet to be discovered may have to be administered prophylactically.

We recall that Windaus had to spend four weeks, waiting impatiently for the results of each one of his vitamin D assays, and can well imagine what it would mean to test each "suspicious" steroid in healthy young people in order to find out—20 years later—whether or not its application has prevented arteriosclerosis. These are the limitations of medicine which only a gifted researcher will someday be able to overcome.

6. Steroids of the Future

A Tentative Prognosis

PRESERVATION OF OUR ENVIRONMENT

Steroid research over the past 50 years represents the greatest concentrated effort ever experienced in the history of the pharmaceutical, and perhaps the entire chemical, industry as well. Never has more time, money and inventive genius been spent on any other group of drugs, and this will probably be the case for a long time to come.

In terms of their very substance, the steroids are more difficult to work with than most other drugs. In addition, there have been unusual problems of raw-materials supply ever since the discovery of the corticoids and the birth control pill.

However, what is, and always will be, truly unique are the conceptual difficulties that have made steroid research such a fascinating field. The idea of antibiotics, for instance, once developed—both in regard to procurement of raw materials and application of the drug—could continue following the same proven pathways. The steroids, however, are bodily substances, closely interwoven with vital regulatory functions which generate new challenges and new solutions daily. Through them, we have a way to control over tens of thousands of cell activities, most of which we are not even aware of.

No matter how much these facts serve to stimulate the imagination of chemists, biologists and physicians, none of them are able to tell us where this journey is headed. Asked about the future, Selye comments: "People always imagine these things to be so easy. Take, for instance, the work with the catatoxic steroids . . . it did not progress in accordance with an overall plan. It is only through the wisdom of *hindsight* that we can identify the steps that eventually led to this concept."

It is, therefore, risky to make any predictions. Nevertheless, one thing is certain: the steroids can never be replaced in the therapeutic repertory. Their mechanism is too closely related to the very processes of life. In a certain sense, they represent terminal points of biological research beyond which we cannot go. In some areas it will be possible to penetrate to greater depths for another 20 or 30 years, for example, with regard to cancer. In other fields, such as insect control, growth will soon mean branching out.

It is very difficult to advance a prognosis, but the future of steroids will probably be based on three of their most salient properties: their capability of penetrating cell membranes with ease, their unique influence on DNA, and—last, but not least—their susceptibility to detoxification in a body adapted to them for millions of years.

We have already indicated what is still needed: further illumination of the ends of the spectrum and isolation of individual wavelengths and, above all, development of filters. Given these prerequisites, some short-term goals are beginning to take shape which fall within the scope of the great objectives of medicine: preservation of our environment, expansion of the therapeutic repertory and the fight against cancer.

As far as preservation of our environment is concerned, as recently as the turn of the century, no one would have counted the restriction of life among the goals of medicine. However, since then, the time mankind takes to double its numbers has dropped drastically—from 70 to 30 years. Within 30 years, there will be 7 billion people on this earth; within 60 years, 15 billion; and within 90 years, 30 billion. In other words, within a time span less than the one that separates us from Darwin, we will be facing catastrophe. The steroids have shown us the first fixed point for applying some leverage against this destructive proliferation.

This means that the application of steroids in the control of population growth will have to increase, since they are much more effective than any other means of contraception. Science will develop steroids that will be virtually without side-effects, and once the realization of their necessity has sunk in, thousands of factories will have to produce billions of birth control pills daily. Perhaps, by that time, instead of pills, we will have monthly injections or additives to bread (with occasional counter-hormones to neutralize their effect), but the drugs assigned to this task will be steroids.

Simultaneously, it will be necessary to ensure the food supply for human beings, who will be competing for this food with rivals that had been considered eliminated long ago.

We believe that we are the rulers of this earth because we are responsible for the eradication of the giant whales, the ferocious tiger, the condor in the Andes. Four billion humans against 5000 tigers—some heros! However, what about an enemy that has us outnumbered? What if we were to consider insects—of which, according to Carrol Williams, 300 million compete with each individual one of us, and of which there are more species than all plants and animals put together?

Now, where is our dominance? Despite modern insecticides, we have been unable, so far, to exterminate even one single species of insect. Although we have broken the genetic code, know how to use nuclear energy, and can travel to the moon and beyond, insects still consume 10% of the crop in the United States, 25% in Kenya and 75% in Tanzania. In the underdeveloped countries, insecticides will soon be more costly than seed grain and fertilizer. The killer bees continue their relentless northbound migration from Brazil. They have reached Mexico, and absolutely nothing can stop them if they have made up their minds to penetrate into the United States.

The estimated septillion insects living on earth, put together, weigh 10 times as much as all humans and hence need 10 times as much food. They move into our homes whenever they feel like it, eat our crops, suck our blood, kill and mutilate our fellow men, transmit malaria, sleeping sickness, onchocerciasis.

For a short while, around 1945, it looked as though we might be able to force them back; first, DDT, then the phosphorus insecticides, were employed on a large scale. Now, however, more than half of all harmful insects have developed immunity to these compounds, and we are faced with consequences we did not bargain for: destruction of many useful animal species and accumulation of DDT, aldrin, dieldrin, heptachlor, and chlordane in our bodies—all of which, we fear, might cause cancer.

Thus far, all of our attempts against the insects have been rendered ineffective by their most efficient form of defense—their frightening fertility. If even 1% of a species remains immune against an insect poison, only a few years are needed for that species to be back to 100%, ready for the next insecticide.

W. J. Holland writes: "When all cities have long since died and crumbled and all life on this earth is almost extinct, there will be a tiny insect, sitting on a lichen patch, extending its antennas into the light of a burnt-out sun. . . ."

Even now, there is no longer any talk about holding back the insects, let alone destroying them. Experts speak of a *tentative* "balance," as though this represented a great vitory. Now that steroids are becoming visible on the horizon, perhaps they will supply the means of maintaining that "balance."

Ever since Karlson's discovery, the idea of using steroids against insects has been an obvious solution to our problem. The advantage of ecdysones is simple: they attack the enemies' strongest point, their fertility. They prevent pupation, or exaggerate it. Besides, no one has ever heard of developing immunity to steroids. Resistance can be developed only via the genes, and any organism whose genes could develop immunity to its own, most vital hormones would probably have become extinct a long time ago. Furthermore, with regard to the toxicity of this particular steroid category to man and animals, luck appears to be on our side: since only arthropods undergo pupation, they are the only ones that respond to the ecdysones. These will probably, therefore, be harmless to other animals. However, the most important property of the ecdysones may be the fact that they cannot accumulate—neither in the soil, where they are destroyed by rain, nor in the body, which is equipped to eliminate steroids.

Initially, the implementation of such an idea encountered great difficulties. The development of suitable substances of this type was hampered by the fact that, until a few years ago, thousands of kilograms of insects had to be processed to recover a few milligrams of these hormones (which must be applied by the ton).

Then, in 1966, Japanese researchers found that some plants contain ecdysone-like steroids which have a strong hormonal effect on insects. Meanwhile, many other ecdysones have been found in plants, in large quantities, so that their utilization as pesticides has moved within the range of possibility.

Besides interfering with pupation, these ecdysones inhibit ingestion of food. Tests performed in Italy have shown that silkworms, feeding on mulberry leaves sprayed with muristerone (an ecdysone), stopped feeding and died soon thereafter (see Fig. 6–1).

Since, moreover, the various ecdysones appear to be specific for particular species, it may even be possible to selectively spare useful species. No doubt, it will take years until these ideas can be brought to practical application, but certainly this will be the next major field in which the steroids will display their abilities, a field whose limits cannot as yet be envisioned.

In addition to safeguarding our food supply against pests, the steroids

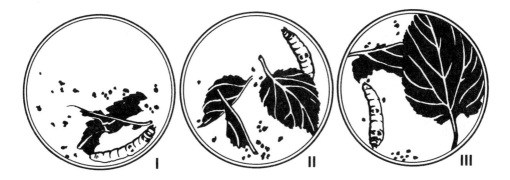

Fig. 6–1. The silkworm, feeding on leaves. Appetite decreases as leaves are sprayed with increased amounts of steroids.

can also help fill our survival needs in other ways, for example, by improved utilization of available food sources. Hormonal improvement of meat through castration had been a known practice even in ancient times. Today, this method has largely been replaced by "chemical castration" which, until a few years ago, was obtained by administration of the inexpensive drug stilbestrol, a non-steroid. Because this substance is not destroyed by cooking or frying, and reports of consequent incidences of cancer ensued, this drug was prohibited in the United States. Ever since, each head of cattle has required, roughly, an additional 250 kg of feed before it is ready for slaughtering. This means that it will be necessary to develop better methods of chemical castration by somewhat more expensive, but harmless, steroids which can be degraded by cooking. This method of "castration" will also have the added advantage that skillful selection of steroids can determine whether the meat is to be soft or firm, dark or light, lean or fatty.

On their way to the slaughterhouse, most animals, because of stress, break down proteins and retain water in their tissues. Thus, the quality of the meat becomes markedly poorer. Steroid blockers could prevent this.

However, this is not all. By means of steroids, milk production can be enhanced. Also, the number of eggs laid per day can be increased without forcing chickens to live degrading lives an egg-laying machines in 24-hour-daylight coops.

Steroids have the capability of controlling fertility—in both directions. The growing nuisance of excessive numbers of pigeons in public places can be controlled unobtrusively, by using steroids to turn corn kernels (which other birds will not eat) into contraceptive pills. In other animals, such as pets or race hounds, it will be possible to delay or eliminate periods of heat by means of progesterone.

Of far greater consequence, of course, is the regulation of sexual activity in animal husbandry. This will allow deliberate scheduling of artificial insemination programs, to increase the number of calves. In this field as well, the future belongs to steroids.

However, merely ensuring the survival of humanity will not be good enough. The human being of the future wants to be free of the many hardships that still burden *our* lives.

EXPANDING THE THERAPEUTIC REPERTORY

Making life *easier*—this means freedom from suffering; it means a dignified old age. The steroids have initiated the first phase of freedom from suffering: the battle against the obvious diseases—rheumatoid arthritis, endocarditis, the entire complex of immunological diseases, including transplant problems—

would not be possible without glucocorticoids; just as the treatment of endocrine disorders would be unthinkable without the sex hormones. Prophylactic measures against rickets, digitalis therapy, and aldosterone blockers have become indispensable.

New uses will be added, as well as improved medications. In 1955, the first steroid was used in intravenous anesthesia; today, we have steroids in which the ratio between effective and toxic doses has been improved from 1:7 to 1:30. In other words, they are four times safter than the usual anesthetics.

In addition, steroids will be used as tranquilizers, pain relievers and anti-biotics. Therapy will take advantage not only of the steroids' hormonal effects but also of their capability of penetrating the cell membrane. Pyrroli-dine, attached to positions C-3 and C-17 of a steroid, penetrates into the cell and induces muscle relaxation, an effect that has therapeutic potential (see Fig. 6–2). Similarly, cardiac-active substances will be attached to steroids to permit transport into the cardiac muscle cell. This will lead to effects that are close to those of the cardiac glycosides and, perhaps, will even surpass them one day. Also, it has apparently become possible to dissolve gallstones in the body without resorting to surgery: by means of chenodesoxycholic acid.

New indications for the treatment of disease crop up every day. Male hormones can reduce the severity of damage in aplastic anemia, as well as in anemia associated with chronic kidney diseases. Female hormones, on the other hand, are employed to stimulate ovulation in infertile women, or as

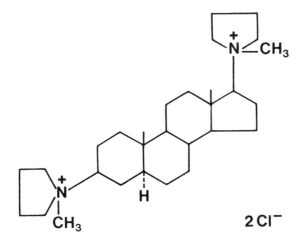

Fig. 6–2. Example of muscle-relaxing molecules, receiving transport help from a steroid.

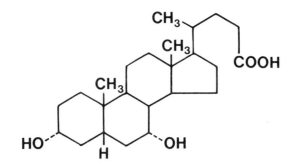

Fig. 6-3. Chenodesoxycholic acid.

antidepressants during menopause. Steroids are used against growth to excessive height, skin disorders, myocardial infarctions, pulmonary fibrosis and pemphigus, an uncommon, but serious skin disease. They can be prescribed in the form of tablets, injections, ointments, inhalations, sprays and eye drops. Today, so many years after Hench's discovery, the list of new indications keeps growing daily, and there is no end in sight.

In addition, chemical research is busy developing new synthetic steroids without side-effects, or with custom-designed concomitant effects. Each individual hormonal property will be available separately, or its excess in the body will be selectively blockable.

Then, scientists will stop to take a deep breath before tackling the second phase, the therapy of chronic and less obvious diseases. The difficulties associated with this endeavor have already been mentioned, as well as the first attempts to influence *hypertension* by means of steroid inhibition. It is also possible to use steroids as therapeutic agents against the chronic *poisoning* caused by the waste products of industrialized countries. Someday we may have no choice but to use catatoxic steroids to immunize ourselves against environmental pollution, as we do against smallpox and typhoid fever, or as we regularly take our vitamins.

Hypertension is surpassed only by one chronic, insidious disease which leads to debility and death. Most of us will develop it as we get on in years, and it will kill more of us than any other disease. Only traffic accidents and cancer come close.

Atherosclerosis (*atheros* = fat), or arteriosclerosis (because it affects the arteries), is not easily defined, although we all feel that we know what it is. Like aging, it is difficult to discern what atherosclerosis consists of and when it starts. Trying to describe it, the pathologist would probably say that it is characterized mainly by deposits of cholesterol on the inner surfaces of arteries, where the large whitish-yellow plaques are the distinguishing marks

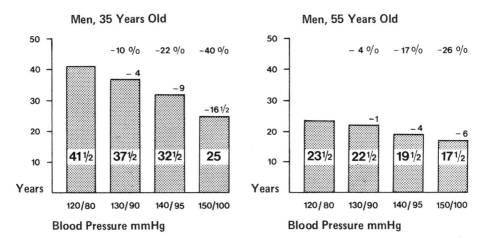

Fig. 6-4. Life expectancy in relation to blood pressure.

of success-oriented western man—at autopsy! The neurologist would probably call it the most frequent cause of senile dementia, something we tend to deplore as "second childhood" in our neighbor (but, strangely enough, never notice in ourselves). The internist, on the other hand, will look at it as the cause of severe hypertension and myocardial infarction, or heart attack.

How these fatty deposits develop is fairly well understood. Cholesterol enters the artery in combination with a protein. Later on, this complex is dissociated: the protein disappears, but the cholesterol deposit remains.

Why this happens in some people and not others is not quite clear. There are some diseases that lead to atherosclerosis, for instance, diabetes and certain liver and kidney disorders. Other people are healthy as can be, but still have abnormally high plasma cholesterol levels. A high blood cholesterol level is in itself a danger signal. In a study of more than 3000 patients, only 1.8% of those with blood cholesterol levels lower than 224 mg per 100 ml (milliliters) suffered heart attacks within ten years, whereas the rate of incidence was 30% for those with levels higher than 375 mg per 100 ml.

Now, what causes such an increased level of cholesterol in the blood? There is no easy answer, but diet plays an important role. For instance, it is possible to produce atherosclerosis quickly and consistently in many animals by feeding them a high-cholesterol diet. When such an animal is examined, the electron microscope shows how cholesterol crystals penetrate the lining of the arteries (see Fig. 6-6).

Consequently, physicians have tried to lower the blood cholesterol level of atherosclerotic patients by prescribing a low-cholesterol diet: no egg yolks, no brains, no calves' kidneys or liver, very little animal fat. However, with

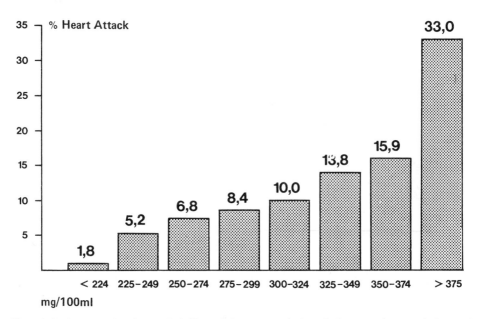

Fig. 6-5. Increase in the probability of heart attack in relation to plasma cholesterol levels.

cholesterol present in almost all animal tissues, the list would be endless. Besides, almost nobody adheres to dietary restrictions.

Therefore, scientists began looking for some means of preventing the absorption of dietary cholesterol. The basic idea was that cholesterol cannot penetrate the intestinal wall without bile acids. Consequently, the trick was to find a way of binding the bile acids in the intestinal tract to prevent their resorption in combination with the dangerous cholesterol. Since, in the test tube, ferric chloride will precipitate bile acids, this substance was fed experimentally to cocks and, indeed, did lower the cholesterol level in the blood. However, the cocks soon died because of the toxicity of ferric chloride. Then, in 1960, Terment discovered a synthetic resin, cholestyramine, which was similar in effects to ferric chloride, but harmless. Harmless? Well, some patients did complain about diarrhea and nausea.

Subsequently, clinicians fell back on another compound that had been known since the thirties: the steroid sitosterol (similar to stigmasterol and other vegetable steroids), ingested along with food in daily doses of 15 g, appears to bind to the enzymes that esterify cholesterol before it can pass through the intestinal wall. We have already mentioned this in connection with competitive inhibition. This prevents the resorption of cholesterol in foodstuffs as well as the resorption of any cholesterol eliminated into the

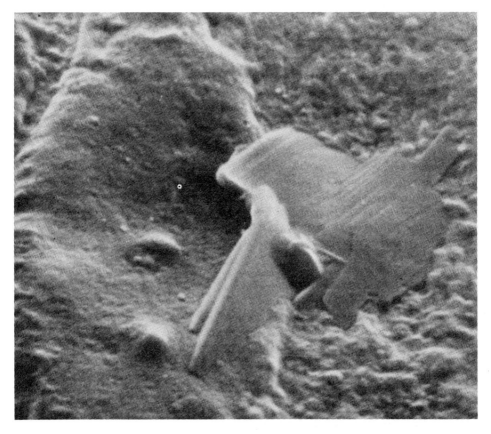

Fig. 6–6. Cholesterol crystal in an artery.

intestinal tract by the body. Absorbed into the body, sitosterol keeps competing with cholesterol for free binding sites in the blood and the tissues—and wins, with the added advantage that, after it has displaced the cholesterol, it is easily eliminated and has no harmful after-effects.

However, it is not everybody's cup of tea to take 15 g of a tasteless substance day after day, and put up with the occasional side-effect of intestinal distress. So, researchers continued to develop new ways of inhibiting the absorption of cholesterol in foodstuffs, starting with ultraviolet irradiation and ending with ingestion of kelp, but people continue to develop atherosclerosis.

Then it was decided to approach the problem by a different avenue: after all, the body produces its own cholesterol, and in such abundance that it still eliminates 1 g each day in fecal matter, even if there is not a single gram in the food consumed. Suppose something could be done to interfere with the

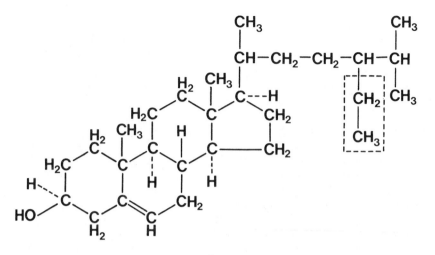

Fig. 6–7. β-Sitosterol.

biosynthesis of cholesterol, which we discussed briefly in a previous section? Therefore, the problem was attacked from this angle—synthesis within the body.

Lynen, when asked why he was working with cholesterol, had a one-word reply: "Atherosclerosis." He feels that the logical way of controlling the biosynthesis of cholesterol is through inhibition of one of the enzymes that catalyze the various steps in synthesis. In his opinion, the enzyme that reduces the precursor of mevalonic acid is the one most suitable for attack.

However, clinical research is nowhere near being able to pick the most favorable place in the body for preventing cholesterol synthesis. One of the first drugs along this line, triparanol, inhibits synthesis at a much later point. Wonderful initial reports spoke of a tremendous drop in blood cholesterol levels. It would have been a very good medication, if one had been willing to put up with a simultaneous reduction in white blood cells and libido, with cataracts and loss of hair, etc.

Other medications were tried, such as nicotinic acid (which causes flushes), d-thyroxine (which may contribute to the development of angina pectoris), or clofibrate (which recently exhibited unexpected side-effects). All of them are effective, but none is harmless enough to permit uncontrolled prophylactic administration to all human beings in the dangerous age category.

It is therefore not surprising that the search continued. Why not try a steroid hormone? Why not pit one steroid hormone against another, as had been done successfully before? The basic consideration here was that women enjoy a relative protection against heart attack prior to menopause, i.e., while they still have their estrogen, but that, later on, they are just as likely to suffer a heart attack as their male contemporaries. Consequently, estrogens were administered on a trial basis—successfully. Unfortunately, however, the amounts of estrogens needed to lower serum cholesterol cause loss of libido, breast enlargement and sterility, side-effects that a man in his forties is certainly unwilling to accept. It is probable that as a preventive measure, a man would have to start taking estrogen at about that age. Later on, it would be too late.

If one turned, instead, to testosterone derivatives, which also lower the cholesterol level, the result was growth of a slight mustache and lowered voice range in women. The hormone approach is obviously quite complicated.

It is strange that something as simple and primitive as cholesterol in the blood is so difficult to conquer. However, this is exactly the challenge that faces steroid research in the future. It must continue to pursue the concept of competitive inhibition, to displace cholesterol (or its precursors) from enzymes by means of specially designed steroids without side-effects, and to reduce blood cholesterol to normal levels (e.g., from 260 to 200 mg). Reducing the risk of a fatal heart attack by a factor of three should certainly be an incentive to scientists.

And should this work be successful, the next problem is just waiting in the wings: nobody thinks that *getting older* is a pleasure either. Or, rather, we should say *aging*. For there is no way of preventing the former, but we can do something about delaying the latter. How?

This is the great question and, in general, researchers agree that it is probably a matter of hormones: not the protein hormones, for their production does not decrease; on the contrary, it is stepped up in order to halt the decline of sex hormone production.

Then, are the steroid hormones involved? Unfortunately, only to a degree. Testosterone replacement therapy in men and estrogen mixtures in women do, it is true, prevent several unpleasant symptoms, but they do not halt the aging process as such. Perhaps there are hormones whose production normally stops at age 20, which would have to be administered from then on to prevent aging, instead of trying to fight it when it is too late.

An alternate theory of aging is proposed by gerontologist Hahn in Basel. He feels that as we get older, the protective proteins which are bound to the DNA of the cell nucleus may turn into a tacky substance which makes transcription increasingly more difficult. Considering this opinion in conjunction with the theory that steroids may produce their effects by removing just these proteins from the DNA, we can envision the possibility of successful research in this direction. In animal experiments, it has actually been demonstrated that enzyme synthesis, reduced in older animals, can be stepped up by steroids. However, to infer that these results may be applied to human beings would be premature. The difficulties inherent in such chronic studies have already been mentioned and appear to be insurmountable for the time being. It is therefore probable that research will turn to more urgent tasks.

Consequently, before scientists tackle the problem of prolonging life, they will first have to fight for its *preservation.* Above all, this means a battle against the deadliest disease of this earth: cancer.

THE FIGHT AGAINST CANCER

Every four seconds, a human being dies of cancer. We know it; newspapers report it every day. Scientists all over the world have been fighting it for 100 years, but there is still hardly anything we can do because we know so little about cancer. Even the terminology is confusing: there are sarcomas, myelomas, leukemias, lymphosarcomas, melanomas, carcinomas, retinoblastomas and many others. These are the names used by pathologists, but they obscure the commonality, the threat, by describing individual aspects instead. To understand the essential nature of cancer, we must ask ourselves: What underlies *all* of these malignant tumors; what makes them so dangerous?

Perhaps the question can be answered in the most general sense by saying that cancer is the appearance of uncontrolled growth in the body, the deviation of a cell group from the coordinated coexistence of the tissues within the organism. Cancer is senseless, merciless growth—until its own death. Whether it ulcerates the skin, destroys the liver, or causes the deterioration of the spinal column, it always starts out the same way. One day, a living cell begins to turn malignant; it proliferates relentlessly in accordance with a law by which it is forced to invade nearby organs by infiltration, to destroy them, consume their nutrients and poison them with waste products.

Thus far, no one has been able to understand this law, although thousands of laboratories all over the world continue to pursue this problem around the clock, simultaneously searching for the causes of cancer and for possible treatments. One fact however, has by now emerged from all this activity: in both areas, the steroids play such an important role that we have reason to assume that they will, some day, help achieve a breakthrough.

In 1932, a connection between cancer and some steroids was probably noted consciously for the first time. In France, with the sex hormones then available in pure form, Lacassagne had induced breast cancer in male mice by the injection of estrogens. At the same time, in England, Cook had been able to produce cancer by means of dibenzanthracene. Three years later, Maisin and Coolen found that methylcholanthrene was 100% effective in producing breast cancer in mice and rats within 4-12 months.

What is the link between these three events? Well, all the researchers were aware of one fact: in 1925, Wieland and others had discovered that the side chain of the bile acids can flip "to the left" and attach to the C-12 atom of the steroid nucleus. Thus, an additional ring is formed between rings C and D; the substance is then called cholanthrene. The notorious methylcholanthrene can also be formed by this pathway, which is shown in Fig. 6–8.

Ever since, scientists have never stopped discussing the possibility that steroids may be capable of turning into carcinogenic (i.e., cancer-causing) substances within the body. This would explain the development of some of the cancers. The Russians in particular, under the leadership of Shabad, have been studying this possibility in detail. They have coined the term "endogenous blastomogenic" to describe those bodily substances that are capable of conversion into carcinogenic ones.

That such a conversion is theoretically possible was shown by Dannenberg of the Max-Planck Institute. However, this man, who is probably Germany's foremost expert in the field, points out simultaneously that it has never been

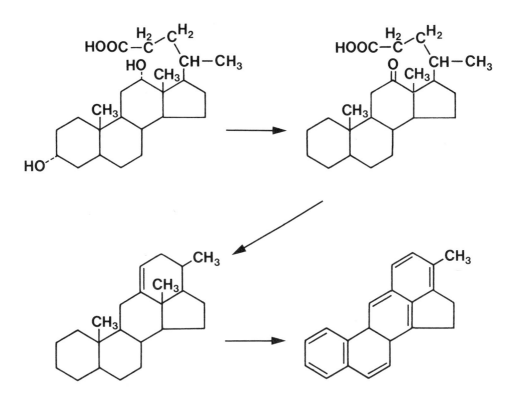

Fig. 6–8. Desoxycholic acid (*top left*), 12-ketocholanic acid (*top right*), dehydronorcholene (*bottom left*), 3-methylcholanthrene, (*bottom right*), carcinogen.

possible to demonstrate the presence of such cancer-causing hydrocarbons as methylcholanthrene or dibenzanthracene in the human or animal body. Accordingly, it appears improbable that the induction of cancer by certain steroids (demonstrated only in animal experimentation) is mediated by their conversion into carcinogenic substances, or that human cancer develops via this pathway. It seems much more likely that steroids, in the extremely high doses used in such experiments, are capable of triggering a predisposition to cancer that exists in the body to begin with.

Among the substances which, next to estrogens, are accused most frequently of being carcinogenic we find cholesterol, which seems strange, because it does not otherwise exhibit any hormonal activity. Not only have oxidation products of cholesterol been shown to cause cancer, but the pure substance as well, dissolved in sesame oil and injected, can induce the growth of malignant tumors in animals.

With a goodly amount of cholesterol and other steroids in our bodies, we can appreciate the dangers we face simply by being alive—without being affected, in addition, by exhaust gases, heavy metals or radioactive waste. However, there is nothing we can do about it. The fact that in order to live, we need substances which trigger cell division, at the same time subjects us to the risk of undesirable mutations. Yet it is precisely this danger that might show us a way out of this dilemma. If we succeed in understanding the processes leading to the development of cancer, then it is also conceivable that we will someday be able to control them. For the moment, our efforts are still empirical, by trial and error. We are still unsure, but some positive results are beginning to appear.

In 1896, a British physician, Beatson, observed that in two women suffering from breast cancer, coincidental removal of the ovaries resulted in improvement. His inference of a connection between the two events was a remarkable achievement, considering that the female hormones were not discovered until 30 years later. Although two cases mean nothing to the statistician, Beatson, with the wonderful clinical-investigative flair of his time, initiated a development which is equally as important as the search for the *cause* of cancer: its *treatment* by means of hormones, or by the elimination of hormonal effects.

At a relatively early stage, much interest was focused on the genital cancers since these involve a direct connection between hormone and target organ. Animal models were needed for detailed studies and, by means of methylcholanthrene, it was relatively easy to induce breast cancer in mice. Moreover, there are many animals that develop spontaneous tumors of the mammary glands. Cancer of the prostate proved to be more difficult. Researchers were unable to produce it experimentally in mice, rabbits or rats. It was the search for a suitable animal model for this cancer that started the ball rolling.

In the late 1930s, Charles Huggins, a surgeon in Chicago, discovered that dogs develop cancer of the prostate. He immediately recognized the importance of this observation in relation to cancer research, and since he was working with steroids anyway, he began testing their effect on cancer of the prostate in dogs.

A white-haired man with old-fashioned, polite manners, Huggins speaks in fluent German: "The most difficult thing was to find sufficient numbers of dogs with tumors of the prostate. Every Sunday morning, my wife and I drove to the municipal dog pound to check out the male dogs: if they had cataracts and bad teeth besides, I knew they were old enough to probably have prostatic tumors. We locked them into the car and took our strange cargo to the lab. Occasionally, we were even stopped by the police, who eyed these trips suspiciously, and I had to make up a story. Anyway, everything went well. We injected some animals with estradiol or testosterone, others were castrated. After some time, we learned that elimination of testosterone (by removal of the testes) or administration of estrogens were the best therapy, and that injection of testosterone caused aggravation.

"Then came the crucial step—application of these findings to the human being. We decided to remove the testes of two patients suffering great pain from advanced cancer of the prostate. It was September 1, 1939!" Huggins says with a meaningful glance. Noticing that this is not immediately clear, he explains: "Two operations were performed for the first time on that day—Hitler's great campaign in Poland, and our insignificant operation in Chicago. As it turned out, ours was to be more beneficial: the operation started at 8 o'clock. Two hours later, the pain had disappeared and our patients already got out of bed. After a few days, the blood levels of acid phosphatase were down. Two weeks later, one of the patients was already playing tennis. . . ."

In mentioning acid phosphatase, Huggins is alluding to a method invented by him, that permits evaluating the effect of prostate cancer treatment after a few days, instead of having to wait weeks to perform X-ray examinations. This is one of the many things that he does not talk about, but that are documented by the numerous diplomas covering the walls of his lab. Since 1958, he has held the German order of merit, and in 1966 he was awarded the Nobel Prize.

These memories are certainly not unpleasant to him, but perhaps they are not as important as the daily morning walk to the Ben May Laboratory, when there is no traffic and the wind blows from Lake Michigan through the grass and flowers. "That is life," he says, "the view of the lake, the trees. . . . And, of course, coffee. Coffee is the blood of the research scientist. Only the human being under our care is even more important. . . ."

Lovable, ironic, that is Charles Huggins, who worked in Germany in 1931, who quotes Dante, Kretschmer and wise Chinese proverbs, and who, incidentally, has given medicine the impetus for hormone treatment of cancer. He raised many questions, but was able to answer only a few—perhaps fewer than he anticipated. For, with time, more and more questions have arisen.

The situation is particularly confusing in the case of breast cancer. In 1942, when Beatson's experiences were generally accepted, surgeons Farrow and Adair asked themselves how, viewed in this light, one could explain the development of breast cancer in women without ovaries, or in men. They removed the testes of male patients with breast cancer and observed a marked improvement. Thus, it appeared that in order to grow, breast cancer needs the male hormone as well.

Since the adrenals also secrete testosterone and estrogens, Huggins and his associates decided, in 1952, to remove the adrenal glands of breast cancer patients of both sexes, whose gonads had been previously removed. Because it resulted in radical long-term improvement, this is the method used today. Naturally, it has to be coupled with adrenocortical hormone replacement therapy in order to prevent the symptoms of Addison's disease.

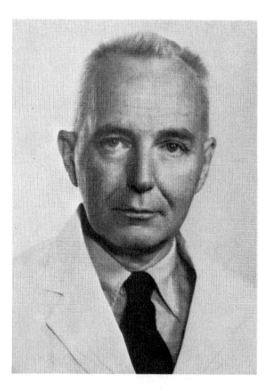

Fig. 6-9. Charles Huggins.

In view of these experiences, there was no longer any doubt that not only the estrogens, but testosterone as well, though they do not trigger breast cancer (or else we would all have it), can support its growth.

To confuse the issue even more, in 1944, Madlow in England found that estrogens can relieve the symptoms of breast cancer, and Huggins obtained remission in over 50% of rats treated with huge amounts of estrogen and progesterone. A few years later, it was demonstrated that testosterone had the same favorable effect in women whose ovaries had been previously removed. Consequently, one had to digest the idea that identical hormones could have absolutely opposite effects.

An explanation of these seemingly contradictory findings is that both prostate and breast cancer are, first of all, products of their organs of origin. As such, they need testosterone or estrogens, respectively. Withdrawal of "their" hormones (or neutralization by administration of the contrary hormone) will inhibit growth of these tumors, until they find a new way of continuing their growth. In this phase, it may be exactly the opposite hormone that is effective. A patient's hormone balance at any given time will determine the direction of these processes and, in modern therapy, the appropriate course of treatment is chosen on the basis of this balance.

We have neglected to mention the steroids of the adrenal cortex; they too show the same ambivalent effect on cancer cells. Breast cancer transplants in mice are more likely to take when the animal simultaneously receives cortisone. On the other hand, some breast cancers, Hodgkin's disease, myeloma and lymphosarcoma can be held in check over extended periods of time by means of high doses of glucocorticoids. This type of cancer is much easier to study experimentally because the diseased cells can be kept growing and subjected to "treatment" in tissue cultures. By this method, it was found that the glucocorticoids are effective even in highly diluted form: an amount of 0.00000003 g per cubic centimeter of tissue culture still kills the cells of certain mouse lymphomas.

From what we have learned, it is obvious that steroid research in the area of cancer has taken but the first few steps along the road. For the future, there are several possible avenues of approach. One involves consistently pursuing the direction indicated by the sex hormones, by developing still more effective substances, or steroid blockers, to neutralize the guilty hormones. This has already been done, for instance, with cyproterone for inhibition of testosterone in cancer patients. Perhaps, one day, surgery can be replaced by "chemical castration," simply by taking tablets.

Furthermore, scientists are busy working out methods of determining the hormonal dependency of a cancer *prior* to the beginning of therapy, thus identifying the hormone most likely to be effective. The underlying logic,

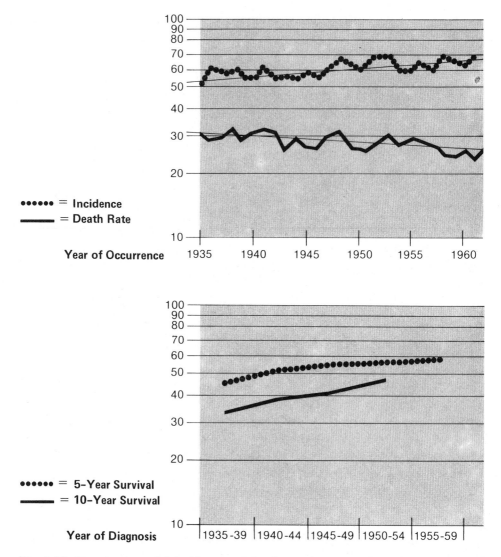

Fig. 6-10. Breast cancer: (a) incidence and death rate (corrected for age) in percent; (b) survival rate (5 and 10 years) in percent.

here, is that a tumor's response to treatment will be more pronounced, the more its cell receptors bind to a certain hormone. Hormones that do not enter the cell will, most likely, not have any effect at all. In order to determine this, the various steroids are labeled by replacing one of their normal hydrogen or carbon atoms with its radioactive counterpart. On its way into the cell, this new atom continuously emits signals in the form of electrons or

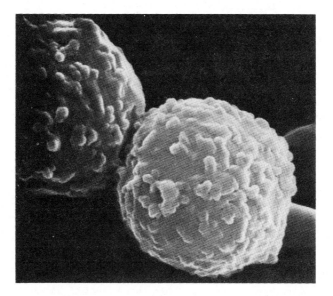

Fig. 6–11. Malignant cell of a lymphosarcoma.

gamma rays, which blacken a subjacent photographic plate just as light does. In other words, from this moment, the steroid carries a lantern which continuously gives away its whereabouts at any particular time. Hormone-susceptible cancer cells will contain distinctly more "black dots" than unaffected cells.

This method simultaneously points toward a possible method of treatment. We can envision the steroid being rendered even more intensely radioactive. Injected into the blood, its molecules would be picked up by the receptors of the tumor cell which would then be destroyed by their radiation.

This development has taken advantage of the steroids' unique capability of locating "their" tissue among the billions of body cells and of slipping through its cell membranes. This same principle has also been used to transport other harmful substances into cancer cells. One of these is nitrogen mustard (similar to the mustard gas of World War I), which destroys the tumor cells. Unfortunately, it also destroys other cells, such as those of the bone marrow. By attaching it to a hormone that selectively enters the prostate cell, its side-effects are reduced and its efficacy increased. Although this too, is just a beginning, the results have been encouraging. A typical steroid of this series is shown in Fig. 6–12. Such a method is obviously not feasible with protein hormones, which have to turn back at the cell membrane and can do no more than activate adenylate cyclase.

In addition to exploiting the steroids' physiological characteristics in this

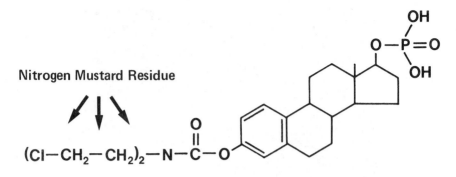

Fig. 6–12. Estramustine phosphate (example of transport help for steroids).

manner, researchers will continue to investigate new steroids, peculiar as they may be. These would include, for example, holothurinogen, which the sea cucumber discharges when attacked, and which kills the cells of a mouse sarcoma in inconceivably low concentrations; or apocannoside from a rare plant which also inhibits the growth of tumor cells.

Another research pathway which, it must be added, is presently the least advanced, might turn out to be the most consequential in the long run: it would attack the cancer systematically at the very site upon which carcinogenic substances produce their direct effect. Huggins, and many others as well, have found that there is a close relationship between cancer-causing substances and DNA, the nucleic acid of the cell nucleus. Recently, this concept has also been confirmed in terms of the virus theory of cancer causation.

This theory states that a virus, the most primitive form of life, consisting of nothing but a nucleic acid core (either DNA or RNA) with a thin protein coat, cannot reproduce without the manufacturing facilities of a fully equipped cell. For this purpose, the virus infects a host organism, for instance with the "flu," by dissolving a hole through the host's cell wall and inserting its own genetic material. This foreign nucleic acid now replaces the DNA of the host cell, forcing it to synthesize nothing but virus nucleic acid and virus protein.

In ordinary virus infections, either the host organism or the virus eventually dies. Sometimes, however, something unusual happens, something uncanny: the viral nucleic acid migrates into the cell nucleus, where it remains latent and becomes part of the cell's genetic material. It is inherited through many generations of cells until, one day, its trait of wild proliferation takes over. Now these are no longer viruses that are multiplying, but human cells. At this moment, a cancer is born.

If we presume that, in the final analysis, steroids act via DNA, then from a

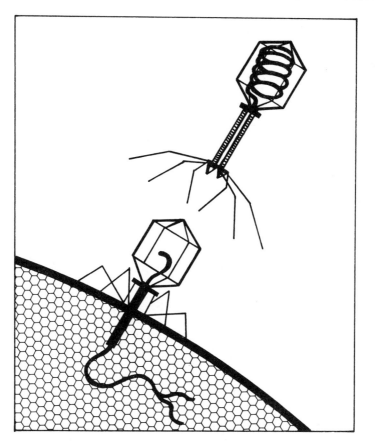

Fig. 6-13. Virus penetrates a cell.

theoretical point of view, such parasitic genetic material should likewise be susceptible to this influence. It is, therefore, not unreasonable to hope that continued research will someday discover steroids which can influence the relatively simple nucleic acid of the virus in the same manner in which they are now influencing the host's DNA. Or one might hope to find steroids that will protect the normal cell in other ways against the effects of carcinogenic substances—by inhibiting activation of the parasitic nucleic acid, and thus suppressing uncontrolled growth, or by stimulating the body's immune defenses. Many scientists believe that all of us are daily producing cancer cells which can, however, be kept in check by natural immune forces. This may be the mechanism which normally functions in the body. On the other hand, this mechanism may only operate in hormonal cancer therapy. There are still too many unknown factors.

Epilogue

The attentive reader may have come to the surprising conclusion that success-ful research is not the result of careful scientific planning. Rather, it depends on a synergistic interaction between human beings of very different natures, brought together by chance. It usually starts with adventuresome thinkers like Berthold, Addison, and Brown-Séquard, who formulate sudden brain-storms into astonishing, frequently still-untestable hypotheses. They are fol-lowed by the inquisitive perfectionists like Windaus and Barton, who develop the necessary test methodology for its own sake. Only when the time is ripe, do the visionary practitioners like Pincus and Selye plant the seed in the pre-pared soil and bring the seedling to maturity with their enthusiasm.

To state it more bluntly: The scientist who sits down and concludes, after some deliberation, that there must be hormones; then, sure of his purpose, proceeds to develop the methodology; and, finally, submits the necessary proof—does not exist! By the same token, no research team has ever sat down and solved such problems by dividing them up among themselves, because one lifetime was not long enough to accomplish everything.

The men who solved the steroid mystery had freedom of choice; they did what they did spontaneously, without planning—perhaps with an eye to fame, but always true to their inclinations.

The necessity for such freedom, then, would appear to be the most impor-tant inference to be drawn from this era in the history of science. At a time when goal-oriented research is being demanded, each page of this book speaks out against such a demand. It is true—only success stories have been reported here, only one out of a thousand crazy hypotheses ever turns out to be fruitful, only a fraction of the esoteric methodology hatched every day finds its way to practical application, and nine out of ten visionaries fall flat on their faces.

However, once success strikes, once the star lights up, the result can be a monument to the creative human mind. Were we to ban the playful, the aim-less, the adventurous from our lives, we would acknowledge the loss of our faith in mankind.

Nobel Laureates

Whose work represented a significant contribution toward our present knowledge of the steroids

1927 H. WIELAND, Munich (1877–1957)
"For his investigations of the constitution of the bile acids and related substances"

1928 A. WINDAUS, Göttingen (1876–1959)
"For the services rendered through his research into the constitution of the sterols and their connection with the vitamins"

1939 A. BUTENANDT, Munich (1903–)
"For his work on sex hormones"

1939 L. RUZICKA, Zurich (1887–1976)
"For his work on polymethylenes and higher terpenes"

1943 E. DOISY, St. Louis (1893–)
Although one of the leading steroid researchers, he received the Nobel Prize "for his discovery of the chemical nature of vitamin K"

1950 P. HENCH, Rochester (1806–1965)
T. REICHSTEIN, Basel (1897–)
E. KENDALL, Rochester (1886–1972)
"For their discoveries relating to the hormones of the adrenal cortex, their structure and biological effects"

1964 K. BLOCH, Cambridge, Mass. (1912–)
F. LYNEN, Munich (1911–)
"For their discoveries of the mechanism and the regulation of cholesterol and fatty acid metabolism"

1966 C. HUGGINS, Chicago (1901–)
"For his discovery of hormonal treatment of prostatic carcinoma"

1969 D. BARTON, London
(1918–)
O. HASSEL, Oslo
(1897–)

"For their contributions to the development of the concept of conformation and its application in chemistry"

1971 E. SUTHERLAND, Nashville (1915–1974)
"For his discoveries concerning the mechanisms of action of hormones"

Formulas of the Most Important Natural Steroids

All animal and plant steroids possess common features which identify them, at first glance, as members of the same family. What they have in common is the steroidal skeleton (also called cyclopentanoperhydrophenanthrene) which consists of four rings designated A, B, C and D. They also have in common the consecutive numbering of the carbon atoms and, in many cases, an oxygen atom at C-3, a remnant of their synthesis from squalene.

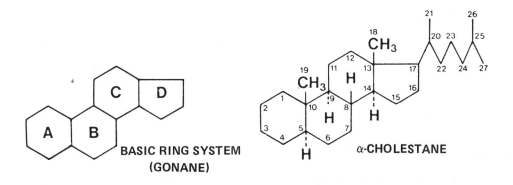

BASIC RING SYSTEM (GONANE)

α-CHOLESTANE

Differences exist in the relative orientations of the rings and substituents (configuration and conformation), the types of substituents, and the total number of carbon atoms in the molecule.

By looking at cholesterol, with its 27 carbon-atoms, as the parent substance of all steroids essential to man, all others may be defined as degradation products. Accordingly, we distinguish between six groups, containing 27, 24, 23, 21, 19 or 18 carbon atoms.

27-CARBON STEROIDS

(a) Cholesterol

This is the membrane component which is probably responsible for permitting the steroid hormones to enter the cell. Moreover, cholesterol is important as the precursor of the steroid hormones.

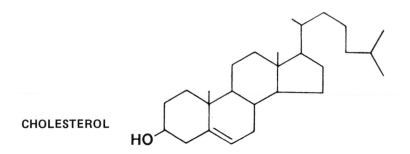

CHOLESTEROL

HO

(b) Provitamin D

An additional double bond (Δ^7) turns cholesterol into a precursor of vitamin D which, by the sun's effect on the skin, is converted into vitamin D_3 (with the B-ring opened up).

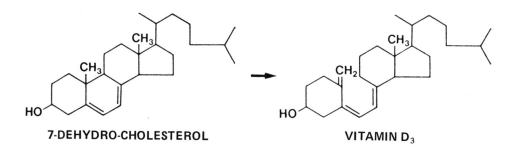

7-DEHYDRO-CHOLESTEROL   VITAMIN D_3

(c) Ecdysone

This distinctly different molecule is found only in the arthropods (and plants). In addition to the oxygen atom at C-6, we notice the extraordinary architecture of the molecule: the methyl group at C-21 and the hydroxyl group at C-14 (which otherwise is present only in the glycosides), as well as the entire A ring, are oriented toward the rear!

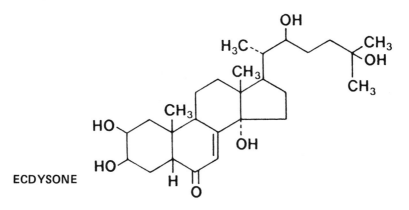

ECDYSONE

24-CARBON STEROIDS

In the vertebrates, specific effects begin to appear in this group. The B ring no longer has any double bonds, and the first degradation of the long side chain at C-17 has taken place.

(a) Bile Acids

The –COOH substituent at C-24 turns this group of substances into the only natural steroid acids of any significance. The three most important ones differ in the number of hydroxyl groups at C-7 and/or C-12. The A ring is oriented toward the rear of the molecule.

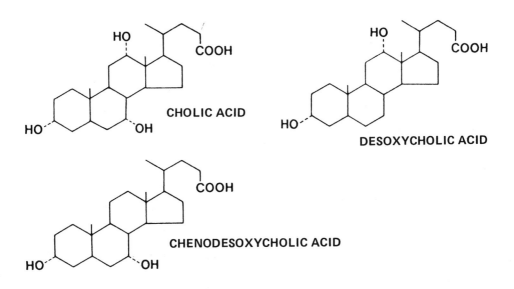

CHOLIC ACID

DESOXYCHOLIC ACID

CHENODESOXYCHOLIC ACID

(b) Bufadienolides

These are the toad venoms, almost all of them highly cardiac-active. Because they are bound to a sugar, they are usually combined with the cardenolides of the digitalis group (see below) in the category of glycosides. The distinguishing feature of this group of substances consists in closure of the chain at C-17 to form a so-called lactone ring. Also typical is the hydroxyl group at C-14 and the rear orientation of rings A and D.

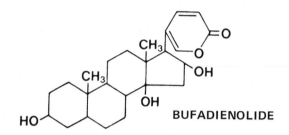

BUFADIENOLIDE

23-CARBON STEROIDS

The degradation continues. Conversion of the six-membered ring at C-17 into a five-membered one turns the bufadienolides into cardenolides. The specific effect on the heart is retained. Most of our therapeutic heart drugs come from this group.

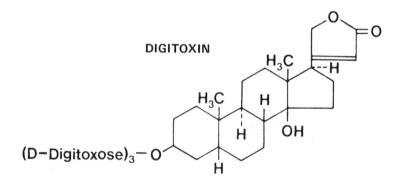

DIGITOXIN

21-CARBON STEROIDS

These start the series of vertebrate hormones. In addition to the corpus luteum hormones, this group includes all of the adrenocortical hormones. The chain at C-17 is reduced to two carbon atoms, and their hormonal activity depends on an oxygen atom at C-20. The prototypes of this group usually possess a double bond in ring A (Δ^4) and the oxygen at C-3 is frequently present in the form of a ketone group (=O) instead of a hydroxyl group.

(a) Corpus Luteum Hormones

Progesterone and its degradation product, pregnanediol, with their oxygen at C-20, are typical representatives of the 21-carbon steroid series. Hormones of this group are collectively called progestogens.

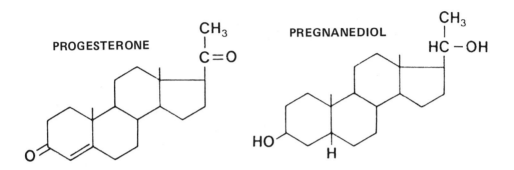

(b) Adrenocortical Hormones

An additional oxygen at C-21 (and perhaps at C-11) results in corticoid activity, influencing mineral and sugar metabolism.

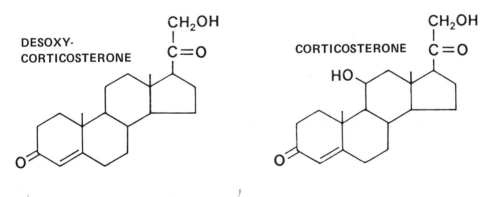

To a certain extent, this effect may be separated into its components. An additional hydroxyl group at C-17 turns these compounds into typical *gluco-corticoids,* primarily influencing the body's carbohydrate balance:

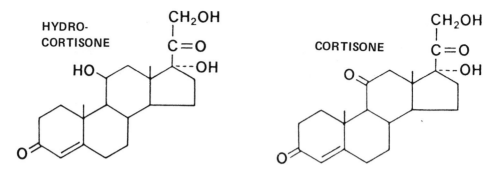

On the other hand, an oxygen at C-18 turns them into highly potent mineral-ocorticoids, influencing the sodium and potassium balance:

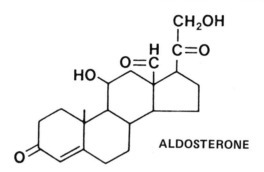

19-CARBON STEROIDS

While the new oxygen at C-17 is retained, the last remnant of the side chain is degraded. This results in the *androgens* group, with their most potent representative, testosterone.

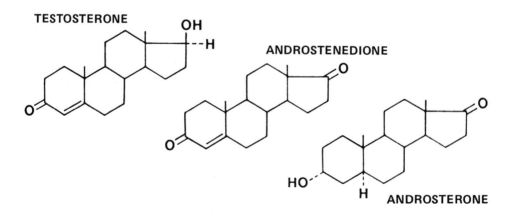

18-CARBON STEROIDS

Elimination of the C-19 atom (which had been attached to C-10) leaves the minimum number of carbon atoms found in physiological hormones. This group is known as the *estrogens.* By means of additional double bonds, ring A is protected against puckering which may result in three-dimensional adaptation to certain receptor molecules. Accordingly, the ketone group at C-3 is converted to a hydroxyl, since C-3 no longer has two arms available for holding on to a ketone. The names of the hormones change according to the number of hydroxyl groups. Estradiol is the most potent hormones of this group.

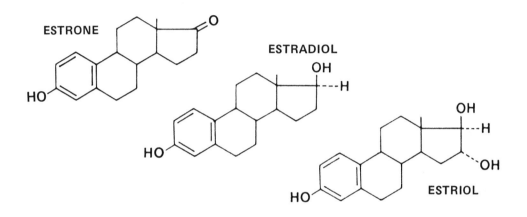

Glossary

Abélard, Peter: 1079–1142, famous scholastic philosopher, born near Nantes, France. After birth of a son and the secret marriage to Héloise, her uncle Fulbert took revenge by having Abélard emasculated.

Acromegaly: Disease caused by a hypophyseal tumor, marked by enlargement of fingers, toes, nose and chin. By affecting the anterior lobe of the hypophysis (q.v.), the disorder may lead to disturbances in the production of sex hormones and corticosteroids.

ACTH: Adrenocorticotropic hormone. From the anterior lobe of the hypophysis. Protein hormone controlled by the CRF (q.v.) of the hypothalamus. Stimulates the adrenal cortex (*see* Adrenal gland) to produce corticoids, in particular glucocorticoids.

Adaptation diseases: *See* Diseases of adaptation.

Addison's disease: Named for physician Thomas Addison (1793–1860). Insufficiency of the adrenal cortex, associated with marked fatigue, bronze coloration of the skin, low blood pressure and sugar. Frequently caused by tuberculosis, or cause unknown.

Adenoma: A benign tumor of a gland.

Adenyl cyclase: Enzyme in the cell membrane which is stimulated by hormones binding to specific receptors, and generates energy and cAMP (q.v.) by conversion of ATP.

Adrenal glands: Endocrine glands which lie just above the kidneys, but are independent of them. Consisting of the medulla which produces adrenaline and the cortex which produces the corticosteroids.

Adrenaline or epinephrine: First hormone to be produced in pure and synthetic forms. Secreted in the adrenal medulla. Effects include increase in pulse rate and blood pressure. No connection with the steroids.

Allergy: Exaggerated reaction of the body to certain substances such as pollen (hay fever), dust (asthma), etc.

Alpha side: A molecule's rear side which binds to an enzyme.

Amino acids: Nitrogen-bearing building blocks of proteins. They are levorotatory (q.v.). Their sequence determines the properties of the protein molecule.

Amorphous: Uncrystallized form of a substance.

cAMP: More accurately called cyclic $3',5'$-adenosine monophosphate. Released through the activity of adenylate cyclase, cAMP acts as a "second messenger," stimulating various processes within the cell, as well as the production of steroids.

Anabolic: Metabolically constructive. Contrary of catabolic (q.v.). Anabolic drugs are substances which stimulate growth, strength, weight gain, etc. Mostly, they are steroid hormones.

Androgens: Substances that stimulate development of male characteristics. Secreted in the testes, ovaries and adrenal cortex. The most potent natural androgen is testosterone.

Angiotensin: Angiotensin I, formed by the action of renin (q.v.) from angiotensinogen of the liver, is converted in the lungs to angiotensin II which, in turn, stimulates secretion of aldosterone.

Anterior lobe of the hypophysis: Site of production of the gonadotropins, ACTH, etc.

Antibiotics: Substances produced by various organisms (bacteria, molds), whose activity is directed against disease-producing germs.

anti fusion: Also called *trans* fusion. Fusion of two cyclohexane rings by formation of equatorial-equatorial bonds (cf. *syn* fusion).

Aplastic anemia: A form of anemia due to damaged bone marrow (benzene, Pyramidon, X-rays, etc.). Sometimes occurring without known cause. Always life-threatening.

A ring: The first ring of a steroid (as compared to rings B, C and D).

Aristotle: Greek philosopher, 4 B.C., keen observer of natural phenomena.

Arrow poisons: Plant extracts used as poisons. In addition to steroids, these include curare.

Arteriosclerosis or atherosclerosis: "Hardening of the arteries." Degeneration of arteries, i.e., loss of elasticity and narrowing of arterial channels. Marked by deposit of cholesterol crystals in the arterial walls.

Asthma: More accurately: bronchial asthma. Brief attacks of highly labored breathing caused by spasms of the fine bronchial ramifications. Usually, it has an allergic basis.

Atom: Smallest, indivisible particle of a chemical element, such as hydrogen (H), carbon (C), and oxygen (O). Several atoms form a molecule.

Axial: Oriented vertically in relation to the (steroid) molecular plane (cf. Equatorial).

Bacteria: One-celled microorganisms that differ from animal and vegetable cells by the absence of a nuclear membrane and sexual characteristics. Only a few kinds are disease producing (streptococcus, staphylococcus, spirochetes). Also important as producers of antibiotics and enzymes which catalyze chemical reactions that would otherwise be impossible, such as the formation of double bonds in the steroid molecule.

Barbasco: Plant of the lily family, whose tuberous roots are particularly rich in steroids. Important raw material source, native in Mexico. Gradually becoming extinct due to excessive harvesting.

Basal temperature: Body temperature of a woman prior to rising in the morning. The temperature increases after monthly ovulation due to release of progesterone. Useful in determining the infertile period in the "rhythm method" of contraception.

Bile acids: Mostly found as "conjugated bile acids," i.e., combinations of a bile acid (a steroid) and an amino acid. The most important bile acids are cholic acid, desoxycholic acid, chenodesoxycholic acid and lithocholic acid—steroids that are indispensable to the process of digestion.

Bohr's planetary model: Named for Danish physicist Niels Bohr, 1885–1962. Atomic model according to which electrons move in orbits around the nucleus, consisting of protons and neutrons, like planets orbiting the sun.

Bronzed-skin disease: *See* Addison's disease.

Buffalo-hump: Like moon face, often a symptom of corticoid overdosage. The reason for this localized fat accumulation is unknown.

Cancerogen: *See* Carcinogen.

Capon: Castrated male chicken. Comparable to steer, gelding, etc.

Carbohydrates: Sugar, flour, starch. In addition to proteins and fats, this is the third major group of foods.

Carcinogen: Also called cancerogen. Cancer-causing substance (*also see* Dimethylbenzanthracene).

Castration: Removal of the male (or female) gonads. Affects the entire body due to absence of sex hormones.

Castrato choir: Medieval boys' choir. Soprano and contralto voice ranges were preserved by castration.

Catabolic: Relating to the destructive part of metabolism (cf. Anabolic).

Cataract: Opacity of the lens of the eye.

Cerebral sclerosis: More accurately called arteriosclerosis of the brain.

Cholinesterase inhibitors: Substances which prevent the degradation of acetylcholine, thus causing prolonged and uncontrollable muscle contractions. Effective in minute quantities, they are used in therapy, e.g., in the treatment of glaucoma (q.v.) and in warfare as so-called nerve poisons (Tabun, etc.).

Chromosomes: DNA strands in the cell nucleus. Carriers of genetic material. Human beings have 23 pairs of chromosomes: 22 pairs of so-called autosomes and one pair of sex chromosomes (XX or XY).

Circadian: Involving a rhythm of approximately 24 hours.

cis **fusion:** *See syn* fusion.

Cloaca: Common opening for intestinal and urinary discharge.

Conn's disease: Adrenocortical tumor named for American physician Jerome Conn. Over-production of corticosteroids, particularly aldosterone, leads to hypertension and loss of potassium.

Contraception: Prevention of conception. Fertilization of the ovum is preventable by various methods. Hormonal contraception is the most effective one.

Copernicus: Astronomer, 1473–1543. Established that the sun is the center of our planetary system.

Cortex: Outer layer, as in "adrenal cortex." Derivatives: corticoids, cortisone, etc.

Corticoids: Steroids having adrenocortical hormone activity.

Corticosteroids: Hormones of the adrenal cortex and their metabolites. They have 21 carbon atoms and are generally distinguished as glucocorticoids and mineralocorticoids. Origin notwithstanding, the small amounts of sex hormones produced in the adrenal cortex are not considered corticosteroids.

CRF: Corticotropin-releasing factor. Hormone of the hypothalamus which stimulates the production of ACTH in the hypophysis and thus, indirectly, the secretion of cortico-steroids.

Cushing's disease: Named for American surgeon Harvey Cushing (1869–1939). Tumor of the anterior lobe of the hypophysis which, in contrast to acromegaly, leads to over-production of ACTH and, in turn, of corticosteroids. Marked by moon face, buffalo-hump, osteoporosis, impaired potency, hypertension.

Cybele: Phrygian goddess. Her priests and followers practiced emasculation to serve the goddess.

Cytoplasm: All the protoplasm of a cell between the nuclear membrane and the cell wall.

Dehydrogenate: To remove hydrogen from a molecule. The resultant substances are identified by the prefix "dehydro-", as in dehydrocholesterol.

Deoxidation: Removal of oxygen from a molecule. The resultant substances are identified by the prefix "deoxy-" or "desoxy-", as in desoxycholic acid.

Dextrorotatory: Rotating the plane of polarization of light to the right (cf. Levorotatory).

Diabetes: More accurately, diabetes mellitus (= honey-sweet). Marked by excessive amounts of sugar in the blood resulting from insufficient secretion of insulin by the pancreas.

Diffusion: Process whereby adjacent liquids or gases slowly intermingle, based on move-ment of the molecules due to thermal agitation.

Digitalis: Foxglove plant whose two varieties *purpurea* and *lanata* supply important cardiac drugs. They are glycosides, i.e., combinations of a steroid with several sugar molecules, such as digitoxin. The steroid as such is identified by the suffix "-genin," as for instance in digitoxigenin.

Dimethylbenzanthracene: Most potent representative of a group of carcinogenic sub-stances which are structurally related to the steroids. Also in this group are methylchol-anthrene, dibenzanthracene, etc.

Dioscorea: Plant of the order Liliales, whose roots are a raw-materials source for steroid synthesis.

Dioscorides: Emperor Nero's Greek physician who traversed the world with the Roman armies during the first century A.D. He compiled what was known at the time about therapeutic agents in his *De materia medica* which, in the Orient, is still consulted even today.

Diseases of adaptation: Term coined by Hans Selye to describe exaggerated reactions of the body (*see* Stress).

DNA: Deoxyribonucleic acid. Long, double-helical molecules in the cell nucleus. They are made up of an almost endless sequence of nucleotides (each consisting of a base, a sugar and a phosphate unit). They are the chemical basis of heredity: transcripts of specific individual DNA strand segments provide the instructions for assembly of specific enzymes.

DOC: Desoxycorticosterone, also called cortexone. Precursor of aldosterone. The first corticosteroid to be synthesized.

Doping: Administration of performance-enhancing drugs to athletes. Frequently, anabolic drugs are used for building up muscle protein.

Edema: Accumulation, in body tissues, of watery fluid lost from the blood vessels.

EKG: Electrocardiogram. Written record of electrical processes occurring during heart muscle activity and measured by an electrocardiograph. These electrical events are extremely sensitive indicators of abnormalities.

Electrolytes: Electrically charged molecules or ions in solution.

Embryo: The developing human individual in the uterus prior to formation of organs, approximately during the first three months of pregnancy (cf. Fetus).

enantio-steroids: Steroids possessing mirror-image structure, mostly without biological activity, probably because they do not "fit" into the enzymes.

Endocrine: Internally secreting. Relating to ductless glands which secrete hormones into the blood (rather than into an external duct).

Endometrium: The mucous membrane lining the uterus. Under the influence of estrogens and progestogens, it causes monthly bleeding or permits implantation of the fertilized ovum, respectively.

Endoplasmic reticulum: The cell's equipment for the production of enzymes. It includes ribosomes and microsomes.

English disease: *See* Rickets.

Enzymes: Complex proteins that reduce the energy required for biological reactions, many of which could not occur in their absence. They control all the chemical reactions in the body and are produced on the ribosomes of the cell (biological catalysts).

Equatorial: Oriented within the plane of the steroid molecule (cf. Axial).

Esoteric: Understood by the specially initiated alone.

Ester: Salt formed predominantly by the reaction between an organic acid and an alcohol. The most important method of salt formation in the body.

Estrogens: Substances exhibiting estradiol-like effects.

Eunuchs: Castrated harem guards.

Evolution: In contrast to revolution, a slow process of development under the influence of natural selection.

Fetus: The unborn child in the uterus, after formation of organs (cf. Embryo).

Fluorination: Introduction of a fluorine atom into a molecule.

Flux: Continuous flow of a stream along a natural gradient.

Folic acid: An essential vitamin of the B complex.

Foxglove: *See* Digitalis.

FSH: Follicle-stimulating hormone. A gonadotropin, secreted by the anterior lobe of the hypophysis, stimulating growth of the ovum and production of sex hormones. In the testes, it stimulates the formation of spermatocytes.

Fungi: Cells which differ from plants by the absence of chlorophyll, and from bacteria by the presence of nuclear membranes. Very few fungi are pathogenic agents.

Gallstone: A calculus formed in the gall bladder due to disturbances in the colloid system; frequently contains cholesterol.

Genin: Steroid component of a glycoside.

Gestagens: *See* Progestogens.

Glaucoma: Dangerous elevation of pressure of fluids inside the eye. If untreated, leads to destruction of optic nerves.

Glucocorticoids: Corticoids whose activity is directed mainly toward carbohydrate metabolism.

Glucosides: Glycosides whose sugar component consists of glucose.

Glycogen: Animal carbohydrate, present particularly in muscle tissue and in the liver.

Glycosides: Combinations of various sugars with steroids (or alcohols).

Gonadotropins: Protein hormones (FSH and LH) of the anterior lobe of the hypophysis. One of their functions is the stimulation of sex hormone production.

Halogenation: Introduction of a halogen atom (such as chlorine or fluorine) into a molecule.

Hermaphrodite: According to Greek mythology, a son of Hermes and Aphrodite whose body coalesces with that of a nymph. In modern usage: an animal or plant having both male and female reproductive organs.

Hippocrates: Greek physician, 460–377 B.C., "father of medicine."

Hodgkin's disease: Lymphogranulomatosis. Malignancies of the lymph nodes.

Homeostasis: Stability of metabolism, temperature, blood pressure, etc., against interfering environmental influences.

Hormone: Active substance produced in the body and exhibiting a specific effect on the activity of cells remote from its site of production.

Hydra: According to Greek mythology, a many-headed serpent, each head of which, when cut off, was replaced by two others.

Hydroxylation: Introduction of a hydroxyl group (OH) into a molecule. The resultant substances are identified by the prefix "hydroxy-", as in hydroxycortisone.

Hypercalcemia: High plasma calcium level.

Hypertension: High blood pressure, in rare cases caused by aldosterone.

Hypocalcemia: Low plasma calcium level.

Hypophysis: Pituitary gland (*also see* Anterior lobe).

Hypothalamus: Brain center controlling the hypophysis by means of so-called releasing factors (such as CRF, LHRF). The hypothalamus performs the important function of processing all the information received from various body tissues and coordinating it into one unified signal.

Infarct: An area of dead tissue resulting from arterial blockage.

Insulin: Hormone of the pancreas, controlling carbohydrate metabolism.

Intrauterine: Within the uterus.

Isomers: Quantitatively identical substances which have different properties based on differences in their structure.

Isoprene: Building block of the terpenes and steroids.

JGA: Juxtaglomerular apparatus of the kidney, which monitors the blood volume and maintains homeostatis through secretion of renin.

Leukemia: Incurable and usually fatal blood disease marked by gross overproduction of white blood cells. Frequently called "cancer of the blood."

Levorotatory: Rotating the plane of polarization of light to the left (cf. Dextrorotatory).

LH: Luteinizing hormone. A gonadotropin from the anterior lobe of the hypophysis. In the male, its effects include stimulation of androgen production and, in the female, maturation of the ovum and production of sex hormones, particularly progesterone.

Lymphosarcoma: Malignant disease of the lymphatic system.

Lysosome: Organelle within the cell, containing enzymes.

Melanoma: Pigmented tumor that tends to become malignant.

Menopause: Cessation of menses in the climacteric or "change of life."

Messenger RNA: A form of RNA which carries the information stored in the DNA of the cell nucleus to the ribosomes in the cytoplasm.

Metamorphosis: Transformation of insects from larva to pupa and finally to butterfly, moth, etc.

Methylation: Introduction of a methyl group (CH_3^-) into a molecule.

Microgram: One-thousandth of a milligram; one-millionth of a gram.

Microsome: Part of the endoplasmic reticulum (q.v.).

Milligram: One-thousandth of a gram.

Milligram equivalent: The quantity of a substance that has a weight in milligrams equal to the atomic weight divided by the valence.

Mimicry: Similar appearance in coloration or form of one animal to another or to the surroundings, usually serving as a protection against predation.

Mineralocorticoids: Corticoids, such as aldosterone, that mainly influence sodium, calcium and potassium balance.

Molecular formula: Total number of different atoms contained in a molecule, e.g., cortisone = $C_{21}H_{28}O_5$.

Müllerian duct: Undifferentiated reproductive duct in the embryo which, in the human female, develops into vagina, uterus, etc. (cf. Wolffian duct).

Mustard gas: War gas similar to nitrogen mustard (q.v.).

Mutation: A change in the hereditary material.

Myeloma: Malignant tumor of the bone marrow.

Nanogram: One-thousandth of a microgram; one-billionth of a gram.

Nitrogen mustard: War gas used in World War I. Causes edema of the lungs and skin blistering due to enzyme blocking. Used in therapy against leukemia and Hodgkin's disease.

Onchocerciasis: A disease caused by presence of worms in the body, occurring in Africa and Central America. Spread by insects, it infects about 20 million people. The larvas, attracted by light, migrate from deep within the body into the cornea and cause blindness.

Osmosis: Diffusion through a semipermeable membrane, typically separating two solutions, that tends to equalize their concentrations.

Osteoporosis: Embrittlement of bones due to various causes.

Ovariectomize: To remove the ovaries by surgery.

Ovulation: Release of an ovum after follicle rupture.

Oxidation: Addition of an oxygen atom to a molecule.

Parathormone: Hormone of the parathyroid glands. It controls the production of the final stage of vitamin D.

Parathyroid glands: Glands that produce parathormone (q.v.).

Pemphigus: Blistery skin disease which may take a fatal course.

Pesticides: Agents used to destroy insects.

Phenobarbital: A barbiturate sedative, similar to Veronal.

Pheromone: A scent that stimulates a susceptible organism over great distances. Only few steroids are known in this group.

Phylogenetic: Relating to the evolution of an animal or plant.

Picogram: One-thousandth of a nanogram; one-trillionth of a gram.

Pituitary gland: *See* Hypophysis.

Plankton: Floating minute animal and plant life of lakes or oceans.

Plasma: The fluid part of blood.

Precambrian: Era preceding the Cambrian, about 1.5 billion years ago, when the earth cooled down and the first organic life evolved in the primordial ocean.

P–R interval: The time it takes from the beginning of atrial contraction to the beginning of ventricular contraction.

Progeria: Premature aging. May be artificially induced by steroids.

Progestogens: Also called gestagens. Progestational steroids, such as progesterone.

Prostate gland: A male gland which tends to develop malignancies in the older man.

Provitamin: Precursor of a vitamin.

Pulmonary fibrosis: Abnormal proliferation of connective tissue in the lungs, marked by respiratory distress. Cause unknown.

Purdah: Indian custom of keeping women and children in the dark, secluded quarters of the house.

Reduction: A chemical reaction that is the opposite of oxidation: removal of oxygen and combination with hydrogen.

Renin: Enzyme of the JGA (q.v.), controlling aldosterone production.

Retinoblastoma: A tumor of the retina. Extremely malignant.

Rheumatoid arthritis: Crippling disease affecting the joints and heart valves.

Ribosomes: Minute particles contained in the microsomes of the endoplasmic reticulum. Responsible for synthesis of enzymes.

Rickets: Also known as English disease. Resulting from a deficiency of vitamin D, it affects the developing skeletal system of children and leads to bowlegs, hunchback, malformations of the skull and pelvis, etc.

RNA: Ribonucleic acid. A nucleic acid which is active in the translation of information supplied by DNA for enzyme synthesis.

Rotation: Optical activity exhibited by many biological substances: the plane of polarized light, passing through such a substance, is rotated.

Saponin: Foam-producing steroid complex. Its steroid component is called sapogenin.

Sarcoma: Malignant growth arising from the connective tissue.

Side effect: An undesired effect in addition to the principal effect of a drug. If needed, what was originally a side effect, may be turned into the desired principal effect.

Skoptze sect: Russian sect of the eighteenth century, practicing self-mutilation. Supposedly has some following in the United States to this day.

Somatic cells: Body cells other than germ cells.

Steroid blockers: Steroids that are effective by competitively binding to receptor sites that would otherwise be occupied by more potent molecules.

Steroids: Compounds containing the basic carbon ring structure of the sterols. They include vitamins, hormones, sterols, bile acids and glycosides, as well as saponins.

Sterols: Hydroxylated subgroup of the steroids. Its most important representatives are animal cholesterol and vegetable ergosterol.

Stilbestrol: More accurately: diethylstilbestrol. Non-steroidal estrogen. Suspected of causing cancer in daughters born to women who took this drug.

Stress: The body's identical nonspecific reaction to various stimuli. Its three stages are: alarm, resistance and exhaustion. Frequently also: the stress-producing agent.

Structural formula: A formula indicating the way the atoms are arranged within the molecule.

Syndrome: Complex of symptoms. Sum of the manifestations of a disease.

syn **fusion:** Also called *cis* fusion. Fusion of two cyclohexane rings by formation of one equatorial-equatorial and one axial-equatorial bond (cf. *anti* fusion).

Teratogenic: Causing fetal malformations.

Thrombosis: Blockage of a blood vessel by a blood clot.

Transcription: The transfer of genetic information from DNA to messenger

Transfer RNA: A form of RNA that delivers amino acids to the ribosomes or assembly in accordance with the instructions provided by messenger RNA.

trans **fusion:** *See anti* fusion.

Trepang: Dried sea cucumbers. Chinese delicacy.

Valerians: Medieval sect, practicing self-mutilation.

Virus: Microorganism. Smaller than bacteria and consisting of nothing more than a nucleic acid core and thin protein coat.

Vitamin: Essential nutrient. Cannot be produced by the body.

Wolffian ducts: The old mesonephric ducts of the embryo which develop into the male sexual organs.

Bibliography

The following bibliography is not meant for the expert. Rather, it represents a selection of documents, some of them historic, which will offer the interested layman an opportunity to expand his knowledge in certain fields, either directly or through the sources given therein.

General

Applezweig, N. *Steroid Drugs.* New York: McGraw-Hill, 1962.

Berthold, A. A. Transplantation der Hoden. *Arch. Anat. Physiol. u. wiss. Med.* **16**:42–46 (1849).

Fieser, L. F. *Steroids.* New York: Reinhold, 1959.

Karlson, P. *Kurzes Lehrbuch der Biochemie.* Stuttgart: Thieme, 1970.

Kreig, M. B. *Green Medicine.* Chicago: Rand McNally, 1964.

Labhart, A. *Klinik der inneren Sekretion.* Berlin: Springer, 1971.

Marti-Ibañez, F. *Essays on the History of Medical Ideas.* New York: M. D. Public., 1952.

Selye, H. *Textbook of Endocrinology.* Montreal: Acta Endocrinologica Université de Montréal, 1949.

Tausk, M. *Pharmakologie der Hormone.* Stuttgart: Thieme, 1973.

Cholesterol

Butenandt, A. Zur Geschichte der Sterin- und Vitaminforsch-ung. *Angew. Chem.* **72**(18): 645ff. (1960).

Liebigs Annalen **447**:233 (1926); *see* "Windaus," p. 233.

Vitamin D

Brockman, H. Die Chemie der antirachitischen Vitamine. *Ergeb. Vit. u. Horm. Forsch.* **2** (1939).

Intern. Nephrol. Congr. Mexico. Variationen über Vitamin D. *Selecta* (21 May 1973).

Loomis, W. F. Rickets. *Sci. Am.,* 77ff. (December 1970).

New ideas on vitamin D. *Brit. Med. J.* (17 March 1973).

Bile Acids

Begemann, F. Die Bedeutung der Gallensäuren für die Verdauung. *Med. Klin.,* 1024–1029 (1973).

Dane, E. Die Arbeiten H. Wielands auf dem Gebiet der Steroide. *Naturwissenschaften* **30**:322 (1942).

Wieland, H. *Hoppe-Seyler's Z. Physiol. Chem.* **98**:59 (1916).

Sex Hormones

Butenandt, A. Ergebnisse und Probleme in der biochem. Erforschung der Keimdrüsenhormone. *Naturwissenschaften* (1936).

Clauberg, C. *Die weiblichen Sexualhormone.* Berlin: Springer, 1933.

Haller, J. H. *Ovulationshemmung durch Hormone.* Stuttgart: Thieme, 1971.

Lauritzen, Ch. Vorschläge zu einer gezielten Behandlung mit Östrogenen und Gestagenen. *Z. Ther.*, 65–82 (1964).

Pincus, G. *The Control of Fertility.* New York: Academic Press, 1965.

Protective Steroids

Brower, L. P. Ecological chemistry. *Sci. Am.* (February 1969).

Habermehl, H. Die biologische Bedeutung tierischer Gifte. *Naturwissenschaften,* 15–21 (1975).

Neuwintger, H. D. Afrikanische Pfeilgifte. *Naturwiss. Rundschau* **27**:340–359, 385–402. (1974).

Reichstein, T. Cardenolide als Abwehrstoffe bei Insekten. *Naturwiss. Rundschau* **20**:499–511. (1967).

Schildknecht, H. Naturally occurring steroid isobutyrates. *Proc. 3rd Intern. Congr. Horm. Steroids, Hamburg 1970. Excerpta Med.* (1971).

Withering, W. *An Account of the Foxglove.* New York: Henry Schuman, Dover Publications, 1961.

Cortisone

Hench, P. S. The reversibility of certain rheumatic and nonrheumatic conditions by the use of cortisone. In *Les Prix Nobel.* Stockholm: Norstedt & Söner, 1951.

Kaiser, H. *Cortisonderivate in Klinik und Praxis.* Stuttgart: Thieme, 1968.

Kendall, E. C. The development of cortisone as a therapeutic agent. In *Les Prix Nobel.* Stockholm: Norstedt & Söner, 1951.

Reichstein, T. Chemie der Nebennierenrindenhormone. In *Les Prix Nobel.* Stockholm: Norstedt & Söner, 1951.

Catatoxic Steroids

Selye, H. *Stress without Distress.* New York: Lippincott, 1974.

Solymoss, B. *Proc. Soc. Exp. Biol. Med.* **151**:940 (1966).

Vollrath, L. Umweltbedingte Anpassung und Schädigung innerer Organe. *Dtsch. Med. Wochenschr.* 1563ff. (1974).

Aldosterone

Melby, I. C. Aldosterone inhibitors. In *Clin. Endocrinology.* New York: Grune & Stratten, 1968.

Pellegrini, R. *Un Nuovo Anti-Aldosteronico.* Milan: Collana, 1973.

Simpson, S. A. Konstitution des Aldosterons, des neuen Mineralocorticoids. *Experientia* **10**:132 (1964).

Thorn, G. W. The adrenal cortex—historical aspects. *Johns Hopkins Med. J.* **123**:49 (1968).

Witzmann, R. et al. Extra-renal activity of aldosterone and its antagonists. *Excerpta Med.* (1971).

Evolutionary History

Afanass'ev, A. *Steroide und Mikroorganismen, Ideen des exakten Wissens.* Stuttgart: Deutsche Verlags-Anstalt, 1972.

Barrington, E. J. Evolution and hormones. *Proc. 2nd Intern. Symp. Growth Hormone, Milan 1971. Excerpta Med.* **244** (1972).

Euler, U. S. v. *Comparative Endocrinology.* Vols. I and II. New York: Academic Press, 1963.

Hanke, W. *Vergleichende Wirkstoff-Physiologie der Tiere.* Stuttgart: Fischer, 1973.

Reinboth, R. Experimentell induzierter Geschlechtswechsel bei Fischen. *Verh. Dtsch. Zool. Ges. Munich,* 67–73 (1963).

Tscheche, R. Pflanzliche Steroide mit 21 Kohlenstoffatomen. *Chem. organ. Naturstoffe,* 99–148 (1966).

Hormonal Messengers

Claude A. Villee (ed.) *Mechanism of Action of Steroid Hormones.* New York: Pergamon, 1961.

Clegg, P. C. *Introduction to Mechanisms of Hormone Action.* London: Heinemann, 1969.

Engel, L. L. *Physical Properties of Steroid Hormones.* New York: Pergamon Press. 1961.

Molecular Biology

Barton, D. H. The conformation of the steroid nucleus. *Experientia* **VI**(8):316–320 (1950).

Holland, W. C. *Molekulare Pharmakologie.* Stuttgart: Thieme, 1967.

Krause, R. Indications of pharmacologic activity of newer retrosteroids. *Proc. 3rd Intern. Congr. Horm. Steroids, Hamburg 1970. Excerpta Med.* (1971).

Lambert, J. B. The shapes of organic molecules. *Sci. Am.,* 58 (1973).

Villee, C. A. *Mechanism of Action of Steroid Hormones.* New York: Pergamon Press, 1961.

The Solution

Karlson, P. *Wirkungsmechanismus der Hormone.* Coll. Ges. ph. Chemie. Berlin: Springer, 1967.

Sutherland, E. W. On the biological role of cyclic AMP. *J. Am. Med. Assoc.,* 1281–1288 (1970).

Wilson, J. D. Recent studies on the mechanism of action of testosterone. *N. Engl. J. Med.,* 1284ff. (1972).

Woese, C. R. Evolution of the genetic code. *Naturwissenschaften* **60**:447–459 (1973).

Synthesis

Block, K. The biological synthesis of cholesterol. In *Les Prix Nobel.* Stockholm: Norstedt & Söner, 1965.

Hardman, R. Pharmaceutical products from plant steroids. *Trop. Sci.* **9**:196 (1969).

Lynen, F. Der Weg von der aktivierten Essigsäure zu den Terpenen und Fettsäuren. In *Les Prix Nobel.* Stockholm: Norstedt & Söner, 1965.

Maisel, A. Q. *The Hormone Quest.* New York: Random House, 1965.

Marker, R. New sources for sapogenins. *J. Am. Chem. Soc.* **69**:2242 (1947).

Peterson, D. H. Microbiological transformation of steroids. *J. Am. Chem. Soc.* **74**:5933 (1952).

The Active Spectrum

Fazekas, A. T. Korticosteroidfraktionen menschl. u. tier. Organe. *Med. Welt* **44**:3ff. (1972).

Kappas, A. Thermogenic Properties of Steroids. In *Methods in Hormone Research.* Vol. IV. New York: Academic Press, 1965.

Levine, S. Stress and behavior. *Sci. Am.*, 26 (1973).

Sawyer, C. H. Effects of hormonal steroids on certain mechanisms in the adult brain. *Proc. 2nd Intern. Congr. Horm. Steroids, Milan 1966. Excerpta Med.* **132**:123ff. (1967).

Preservation of Our Environment

Minist. Agricult., Bologna. *Informatore Fitopatologico,* I/1973.

Nakanashi, K. The ecdysones. *Pure Appl. Chem.*, 25.

Overbeek, G. A. *Anabole Steroide.* Berlin: Springer, 1966.

Selye, H. *Hormones and Resistance.* New York: Springer, 1971.

Expanding the Therapeutic Repertory

Bad Sodener Geriatr. Gespräche. Hormone—Parameter des Alterns? *Selecta* (1973).

Dick, W. Pancuroniumbromid. *Der Anaesthesist,* 173–176 (1970).

Dollery, C. T. Enzyme induction. *Brit. J. Anaesth.,* 961–966 (1972).

Godfredtsen, W. O. *Fusidic Acid and Related Antibiotics.* Copenhagen: Matematisk-Naturvidenskabelige Fakultet, University of Copenhagen, 1967.

Joyner, C. The effect of sitosterol administration upon the serum cholesterol level and lipoprotein pattern. *Am. J. Med. Sci.,* 636ff. (1955).

Kovacs, B. A. Naturally occurring anti-histaminics with a steroid-like structure. *Proc. 2nd Intern. Congr. Horm. Steroids, Milan 1966. Excerpta Med.* **132**:1021ff. (1967).

Kronenberg, G. Synthetische Verbindungen mit Digitalis-wirkung. *Naunyn Schmiedebergs Arch. Pharmacol.,* 393–415 (1964).

Pierce, P. E. Mercury poisoning. *J. Am. Med. Assoc.* **220**:1439 (1972).

The Fight against Cancer

Bishof, F. *Steroids and Cancer, Progress of Tumor Research.* Basel: Karger.

Dannenberg, H. Über die endogene Krebsentstehung. *Dtsch. Med. Wochenschr.,* 1726–1732 (1958).

Dellenbach, F. D. Beziehungen zwischen Östrogenen und Karzinogenese. *Fortschr. Med.,* 626–631 (1971).

Huggins, C. Endocrine-induced regression of cancers. *Science* **156**:1050–1054 (1967).

Kotsilimbas, D. G. Cortocosteroid effect on intracerebral melanomata. *Neurology,* 223ff. (1967).

Ruderman, N. B. Use of glucocorticoids in the palliative treatment of metastatic brain tumors. *Cancer,* 298–306 (March 1965).

Shabad, L. M. On endogenic blastomogenic substances. *Neoplasma* **17**(6):573ff. (1970).

WHO. *Evaluation of the Carcinogenic Risk (Sex hormones).* Lyon: Int. Agency Res. Cancer, 1974.

Wilmanns, W. et al. Indikationen zur Anwendung hoher Corticoiddosen bei der Kombinationsbehandlung akuter Leukämien. *Klin. Wochenschr.,* 1191–1197 (1973).

Index